Getting a Good Night's Sleep

A CLEVELAND CLINIC GUIDE

By Nancy Foldvary-Schaefer, D.O.

Getting a Good Night's Sleep
A CLEVELAND CLINIC GUIDE

Cleveland Clinic Press/May 2006

Contact:

Cleveland Clinic Press
9500 Euclid Ave. NA32
Cleveland, OH 44195
216-444-1158
chilnil@ccf.org
www.clevelandclinicpress.org

This book is not intended to replace personal medical care and supervision; there is no substitute for the experience and information that your doctor can provide. Rather, it is our hope that this book will provide additional information to help people understand the nature and diagnosis of sleep disorders.

Proper medical care always should be tailored to the individual patient. If you read something in this book that seems to conflict with your doctor's instructions, contact your doctor. Since each case is different, there will be good reasons for individual treatment to differ from the information presented in this book.

If you have any questions about any treatment in this book, consult your doctor.

The patient names and cases used in this book do not represent actual people, but are composite cases drawn from several sources.

ISBN: 1596240148

Library of Congress Cataloging-in-Publication Data

Foldvary-Schaefer, Nancy, D.O., 1963-

Getting A Good Night's Sleep: A Cleveland Clinic Guide
by Nancy Foldvary-Schaefer.
p. cm.
ISBN 1-59624-014-8 (alk. paper)
I. Title.
RC547.F65 1006   616.8'498--dc22
2006008156

Cover and Book Design by: Whitney Campbell & Co • Advertising & Design

Illustrations by: Joseph Kanasz, BFA & Kenneth G. Kula

Contents

Introduction

We are a culture ever curious about the importance of sleep – yet searching for ways to make the most of our waking hours. Our language is peppered with references to sleep (nightcap, catnap), and popular culture has responded to our lack of sleep with solutions to keep us awake: the coffee-shop revolution (think Starbucks) and a wide selection of energy drinks. Recent research reminds us of the importance of adequate sleep and the untoward consequences of sleep deprivation and sleep disorders on the quality of our lives.

Yet sleep deprivation has evolved into an epidemic of sorts. The corporate world pressures us to conform to rigorous schedules. We over-program ourselves, jamming our days with professional, extracurricular, family, and social activities. We even teach our children to do the same, encouraging back-to-back after-school activities that book their free time well into the evening hours. It's no wonder we are running on empty, building up a sleep deficit as we go through our busy lives.

With this, sleep medicine has grown into an established medical specialty, and more people than ever before are turning to sleep specialists and sleep disorders centers for answers. Today we know that sleep affects virtually all aspects of life and interrelates with many disciplines in medicine. As one of the body's basic needs, sleep is responsible for restoring and preserving our health.

There are more than eighty recognized sleep disorders, and as the field of sleep medicine evolves, researchers are discovering more about sleep and wakefulness in humans and advancing ways to diagnose and treat these disorders. In this book, we will highlight some of the most common sleep disorders in a series of case studies. Through case studies, we'll explore the symptoms, diagnoses, and treatments of seven different disorders. We also make generalizations about sleep that may not apply to all; consulting a sleep specialist or your family physician about sleep concerns is the first thing you should do if you suspect you or a family member has a sleep disorder. Each case – and that includes yours – is different.

Dr. Nancy Foldvary-Schaefer, D.O.
Director, Cleveland Clinic Foundation Sleep Medicine Program
Cleveland Clinic

Chapter 1
Who Is at Risk For a Sleep Disorder?

To achieve the impossible dream, try going to sleep.

– Joan Klempner

John and Barb have shared a bed for eighteen years. He stretches out on the left; she curls up on the right. He unwinds to the droning noise of the 11 o'clock news; she retires with a bestseller. John rarely lasts through the first commercial break before dozing off, but Barb's reading light might burn past midnight if she's reading a page-turner. He falls asleep on his back; she prefers her side.

They've drifted off like this every night, their routine predictable and comfortable.

But in the past year, this nighttime ritual has evolved into a frustrating struggle for Barb. A light sleeper, she now falls asleep next to a snoring engine. Minutes after John's head hits the pillow, his mouth drops open and his labored breathing escalates into a loud purr. Before long, he erupts, blasting like a foghorn. She wonders if he should lose a few pounds. They've been eating out a lot lately.

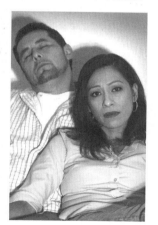

Barb digs her elbow into John's rib and pushes him onto his side.

Huff, puff … purr … snort, snark … choke. He shocks himself awake for a second and rolls back onto his back.

Here we go again, Barb thinks.

She rolls him back onto his side.

John's episodes worsen each week, and when she tells him, "You were really roaring last night," he is surprised. "I was snoring?" It's only when he finds Barb on the couch the next morning that he realizes his snoring is disruptive.

Excuses, excuses

Most of us who complain of sleep problems are armed with excuses for our lack of zzzs.

A worrywart restlessly pores over a mental to-do list. *How am I going to finish this project tomorrow? What did he mean when he said that in the meeting? Am I spending enough time with my children?*

A stubborn professional justifies sleep deficiency as a personality trait. *I've never slept that well anyway. I'm lucky to get six hours.*

Or there's the anthem of the ambitious – more coffee, less sleep. *I'll sleep when I'm dead. Why waste time in bed?*

Chronic nonsleepers chalk up their wakefulness as normal for any "night person." But when we lose sleep, we risk our health. And just as serious are cases of those who sleep all night and drag through the day, exhausted. Job performance drops, they doze off during meetings, and they depend on stimulants to restore their energy so they can spend time with family in the evenings. Sleep disorders affect how we feel both at night and during the day.

And sleep isn't a luxury; it is a necessity. Those hours of lost sleep add up to a greater health deficit than many might realize. We need sleep so we can restore nutrients, replenish the spirit, and refresh the mind. Hidden health hazards accumulate during periods of sleeplessness, and they can't be covered up with concealer or reversed with caffeine.

Sleep ranks in importance with diet and exercise, yet many Americans are sleep-deprived – 70 million of us, to be exact. The number of those with sleep disorders climbs steadily each year, while we continue to regard sleep as extracurricular and optional.

This attitude is dangerous. And sometimes, the side effects from disrupted sleep are extreme.

Take Edward, who hobbled into his doctor's office with a broken leg. His injury wasn't from a sports injury or anything of the kind. The 64-year-old grandfather jumped out of his apartment window while sleepwalking. He was escaping an armed intruder, he told the doctor. Fortunately, he didn't "save" his grandson, who was sleeping soundly in an adjacent room.

Edward's broken leg was a wake-up call to a serious sleep disorder.

After that incident, Edward's wife, Mary, decided that the couple needed a new sleeping arrangement. Now, she tenderly wishes him goodnight in their spare bedroom. Then she locks the windows and door. "I hate doing this," Mary tells him every time.

Four percent of the population sleepwalks, but Edward's activity is more severe than most. Mary compares these nighttime behaviors to those of a werewolf: When Edward is walking in his sleep, he takes on a completely different personality.

A common struggle

Perhaps you aren't like Barb, lying awake at night listening to a snoring bed partner, and you probably aren't mobile at midnight like Edward. But most of us will experience a string of sleepless nights at some point in our lives – times when our minds simply won't turn off and our thoughts race faster every minute we spend watching the clock or staring at the ceiling.

If you're generally a comfortable sleeper, a rare night of fitful sleep gives you a taste of how the other camp copes. You might recognize the morning ritual: The alarm clock squawks way too early, and your subsequent drowsiness and "wrong-side-of-the-bed" mood persist, even after several cups of your caffeine of choice.

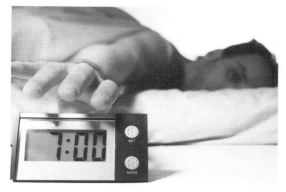

Imagine a week of wake-up calls like this. Or a month. Or a lifetime.

If you recognize this as your morning scenario, you're not alone. Two-thirds of Americans experience frequent sleep problems, according to the 2005 Sleep in America Poll conducted by the National Sleep Foundation. Children, who are as over-programmed and stressed as their adult counterparts, also suffer from lack of sleep. Their restlessness takes a toll on caregivers, who can lose up to 200 hours of sleep each year tending to children's nighttime awakenings, the poll reports.

Meanwhile, not sleeping affects every facet of life: relationships, work, education, appetite, motivation, and more. In turn, certain medical conditions cause sleep problems. Those diagnosed with conditions such as heart failure, arthritis, heartburn, and epilepsy are less likely to sleep well, and overweight individuals are at higher risk for sleep apnea.

It's obvious that we need a good night's sleep. Why then is that so impossible for some of us to achieve? And what is sleep anyway?

Sleep history and mystery

Sleep – what it is, what it is not – has stumped the world's greatest thinkers. Early writers and poets pondered this curious state of being, attempting to decipher its relationship to dreaming and death. Sleep plays starring roles in science fiction as well as the stories we grew up reading – at bedtime, ironically.

Sleeping Beauty was cast under a spell that would allow her to awake from an ageless sleep with a kiss from her true love. Princess Aurora was granted regenerative powers from sleep. Rip Van Winkle rested for twenty years and two days straight. Washington Irving enticed readers with a dreamscape called Sleepy Hollow, where spellbound villagers in the sequestered glen walked in reverie. The Sleepy Hollow Boys, as they were called, heard music and voices in the air, fell into trances, and saw ghosts – like the notorious Headless Horseman.

You can't escape references to sleep. Terminology and slang related to sleep permeate our language: all-nighters, nightcaps, catnaps, night owls, sleeper movies. We are a culture curious about sleep – and, in fact, we've always been that way. We're still looking for answers: What is sleep? And on a scale from awake to dead, where does sleep fall in relation to coma, hibernation, and hypnosis?

Robert MacNish, in his 1834 book *The Philosophy of Sleep*, mused that sleep was a subconscious middleground:

Sleep is the intermediate state between wakefulness and death; wakefulness being regarded as the active state of all the animal and intellectual functions, and death as that of their total suspension.

Sleep puzzled people in prehistoric, biblical, and later times. Dreams, nightmares, and the circadian rhythms of the human body enthralled our ancestors long before science and medicine evolved and research produced data about "normal" sleep cycles (this information wouldn't surface until the 1950s). Distinctions between states of quiescence (coma, stupor, intoxication, hypnosis, and hibernation) were nonexistent. Sleep meant the brain was "off," and when sensory stimulation bombarded the brain, one woke up.

Then the question of sleep flip-flopped.

"It is perhaps not sleep that needs to be explained, but wakefulness," wrote Nathaniel Kleitman in *Sleep and Wakefulness* in 1939. Soon after, scientists studied electrical activity in the brain and discovered clear, repetitive brain-wave patterns – a sleep cycle. Sleep research progressed during World War II to animals, which led to explanations of rapid eye movement (REM) sleep. Sigmund Freud piqued public interest in dreams and sparked more sophisticated studies of brain activity and sleep's relationship with psychology.

Sleep history is steeped in mythology, and the study of sleep and dreams still leaves doctors with unanswered questions. Sleep research has pieced together decades of experiments and debunked historical beliefs of what sleep is, and shown that sleep disorders interfere with wakefulness and are indeed a health hazard.

The basic anatomy of sleep

Why do we sleep? Why do our bodies tell us to take a break so we can refresh, re-energize, and renew?

Bodies naturally maintain an internal equilibrium; this is called homeostasis. Just as our stomach growls when we feel hunger pangs, and our throat is dry when we are thirsty, our body shuts down when we are tired. We have a homeostatic drive to sleep. Our brain tells us when it's time for lights out.

Our "sleep switch" is located in the hypothalamus of the brain; the front regulates sleep, the back is the wakefulness center. However, a variety of other areas within the brain, ranging from brainstem nuclei (collections of brain cells) to structures in the cerebral hemispheres, are involved in promoting sleep and wakefulness. Neurons in these regions interact with each other; some inhibit sleep-promoting neurons during the day, while others collect in the brain during wakefulness and eventually promote sleep at night. This "circuit" within the brain helps the body sustain a sleep-wake balance that is as necessary as food and drink.

Working in tandem with this drive is the circadian clock, which we discuss further in Chapter 11. The circadian clock is regulated by a specific group of brain cells in the hypothalamus. The circadian clock works in sync with the external environment to coordinate sleep and wakefulness.

Together, the circadian clock and our homeostatic drive to sleep tell our bodies when to sleep and when to wake up. Sleep disorders arise when these messages are confused or out of sync.

What We Know About Sleep

Sleep disorders are disturbances that affect normal sleep patterns and wakefulness. There are more than eighty different sleep disorders. Sleep disorders affect everyone, from babies to the elderly, and many who suffer from them do not seek the help they need.

Beyond historical perceptions and mythological hypotheses, the following is known about sleep:

• Sleep needs are genetically determined, and six hours is not enough for most of us. Numerous studies demonstrate that this amount of sleep can negatively affect health.

• We can't learn to sleep less. While some people might adapt to sleep loss, and sleep necessity varies, sleep is a biological function. There is no substitute for it.

• Sleep is not a waste of time. During sleep, a variety of biological processes take place that restore our bodies and minds.

• Sleepiness is not a character flaw. Sleepy people are not lazy or unmotivated. Most likely, they are sleep-deprived or suffer from a sleep disorder and are in need of treatment.

A Billion-Dollar Industry

A quick inventory of over-the-counter sleep aids, products that promise to cure snoring, and herbal remedies indicates that people aren't just talking more about their sleep habits – they recognize that they need sleep and are looking for a cure. Television commercials assure us that we don't have to go another night without it either.

Americans filled more than 35 million prescriptions for sleeping pills in 2004, spending $1 billion, according to National Institutes of Health statistics. Use of sleep prescriptions doubled between 2000 and 2004 among adults ages 20 to 44, according to a 2005 Medco Health Solutions study. More startling is that sleep aid use is up 85 percent among children ages 10 to 19. Sleep drugs are big business, with no sign of lulling into "snooze" as we reach for pill-bottle solutions.

Then there is caffeine, a quick fix for most of us who need a pick-me-up. We turn to stimulants to combat the chronic partial sleep deprivation that modern society encourages. The success of Starbucks is due, in part, to our sleep-deprived society. We demand the strong, caffeinated drinks it sells – and Starbucks sells lots of them.

At the same time, more of us are reserving beds at sleep labs for overnight testing – so desperate are we for a good night's sleep. Today's overnight sleep studies are not reserved just for patients with obstructive sleep apnea. Labs are equipped to test children and cater to those with special needs.

Sleep generalizations

Although men and women share common sleep problems, some problems are more prevalent in one gender than the other. Problems also arise that are specific to teens, children, and the elderly. The following are some sleep generalizations for each group:

Men

General attitudes: *Sleep gets in the way of work … If I'm sleeping, I'm unproductive … Lazy people need more sleep – I've got too much to do and far too many responsibilities … My wife complains I snore like a freight train, but I sleep just fine…*

Sleep obstacles: Some men (and women, too) sacrifice downtime in the evening to work longer and harder so they can get ahead. Rather than reading a book or doing other activities to unwind, they boot up their laptops and plug away into the wee hours. It can take hours to free your mind after an exhausting day at work. Stop number crunching and strategic planning before midnight, and allow your mind to slow down.

In addition to work, men's schedules are packed with home-improvement projects, working out at the gym, participating in sports, volunteering for civic groups, spending time with family, and other personal pursuits. And when life changes enter the picture (like marriage, a new baby, a new job, a move, or a death in the family), men tend to bottle up feelings rather than release them by venting to friends and family. The worry jar almost always opens when the lights are out. And when you can't solve problems, they become more dramatic and urgent, growing from a small "what-if" to a crisis.

When Randy wakes up at 3 a.m. and can't fall back asleep, he worries about his mother, who is in the hospital. He is concerned about job security because his company has been laying off workers, and he is trying to plan a time when his family can go on vacation. All of this goes on in his head until the alarm sounds.

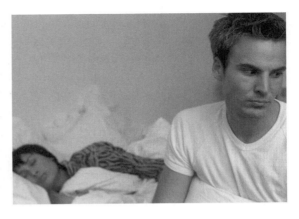

Women

General attitudes: *How can I balance family, work, and friends? ... I feel as if my life is pulled in so many directions, that's all I can think about when I wake up at night ... My body is telling me it needs rest, but my mind won't slow down ...*

Sleep obstacles: Some of the sleep challenges confronting women are related to hormonal changes during pregnancy, menstruation, and menopause. Postpartum depression also triggers insomnia in some women. As a woman progresses through the stages of her life, she is prone to sleeping less or waking up more often during the night. After menopause, women are more likely to be diagnosed with sleep disorders like obstructive sleep apnea.

When Beth was pregnant with her first child, she didn't expect to lose so many hours of sleep *before* she gave birth. But sharp back pain made it next to impossible for her to settle into a comfortable position, and as soon as she drifted to sleep, she had to get up to go to the bathroom. Sounds like a scene from a

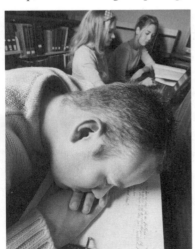

sitcom. But at the time, her aching body and frequent trips from the bedroom to the bathroom were not funny. She found herself napping in the afternoon to catch up on sleep she lost each night.

Teenagers

General attitudes: *With school, friends, and sports, I don't have time to sleep ... I have to wake up for school so early, but I'm not ready to go to bed early at night – it's so hard to stay awake during class ... I'm a night person ...*

Sleep obstacles: Time might be teenagers' greatest challenge, and sleep loses out to school, sports, jobs, and social activities. A recent survey by the American Academy of Sleep Medicine shows that only 15 percent of teenagers get the nine hours of sleep they need each night on a regular basis. That means 85 percent of 13- to 19-year-olds are running on empty. Twenty-six percent of young people clock six or fewer hours under the covers each night.

As the teenage body works through puberty, it also experiences a shift in circadian rhythm (the body's twenty-four-hour clock). Although younger children are apt to feel tired at 8 or 9 p.m., teens' circadian clocks shift to a later sleep time – 10 or 11 p.m. Meanwhile, school starts early in the morning followed by extracurricular activities that carry on late into evening. Sleep is just another elective.

Children and the elderly

Without adequate sleep, a healthy, happy baby can grow into a problem child. A child's disposition often is the first indication of sleep deficit. Rather than being lighthearted, smiling, and energetic, a tired child is cranky and hyperactive.

As people age, their sleep habits change significantly. For those over 65, it is important to distinguish between what is normal and what symptoms are signs of a sleep disorder. Both age groups will be covered more thoroughly in Chapter 12: Sleep in Special Populations.

Chapter 2
Do You Have a Sleep Disorder?

A ruffled mind makes a restless pillow.

– Charlotte Brontë

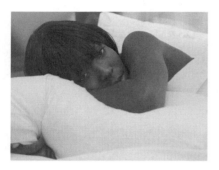

Plenty of exhausted people downplay restless nights and drowsy days by attributing sleep loss to environmental distractions. Take Ruth, who tunes into every drip from the faucet, every creak and curious noise. Each tempts her from her bed to check out what could be causing such a racket. While tossing and turning, she creates a mental to-do list that keeps her up even later. She eventually falls asleep right before her alarm clock buzzes. Does Ruth suffer from lack of sleep? Sure, she says, blaming her tired eyes on noisy distractions.

Or perhaps you can relate to Les, who crashes into a sleep so deep that the blaring television is his lullaby. Nothing wakes him – not ringing phones, cacophony from the living room, or the 110-pound hound dog that joins him in bed as soon as he crawls under the sheets. Yet Les is chronically sleepy most days, regardless of how hard and long he sleeps at night. If he could curl up on a couch between meetings at the office, he'd fall fast asleep. In fact, that's how he spends most Sundays.

These two scenarios are normal to many people. Les and Ruth might remind you of a spouse or even yourself. And though your symptoms might not match theirs or be nearly as severe, the fact that you suffer through long, tiring days is reason enough to talk to your doctor.

Is it a sleep disorder?

How do you know whether your wide-awake nights or sleepy days require treatment from a doctor or sleep medicine specialist? Answering these questions can help you determine whether your sleep habits require attention:

- Are you often tired or sleepy during the day?

- Do you snore or have interrupted breathing during sleep?

- Do you kick or thrash in your sleep?

- Do you have trouble falling or staying asleep?

- Do you have a family history of sleep disorders?

- Do you have unusual sensations in your legs at night that interfere with your ability to fall asleep?

- Do you experience unusual behaviors in sleep such as walking, eating, or acting out dreams that interfere with sleep quality or have caused injury to yourself or others?

- Do you have irregular or inconsistent sleep and wake-up times? Is your bedroom environment noisy, bright, or uncomfortable?

- Has your sleep problem been present for more than three months?

If you answer yes to any of these questions, the night moves you've grown used to and eventually accepted as "normal" are potential symptoms of a sleep disorder. The good news: With monitoring and treatment, you could be able to say "good night" – and mean it.

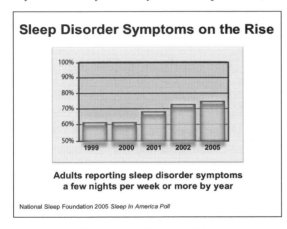

Sleep Disorder Symptoms on the Rise

Adults reporting sleep disorder symptoms a few nights per week or more by year

National Sleep Foundation 2005 *Sleep In America Poll*

First, understand that loss of sleep is not just a nighttime problem. Sleep is designed to rejuvenate the body so it can function properly during waking hours. Your sleep "activity" is just as critical as your daytime activity. The quality time you spend working through various stages of the sleep cycle is just as important to your physical well-being as eating your veggies and taking 10,000 steps a day for exercise. In addition, sleep loss poses an increased risk for certain ailments, such as metabolic and endocrinological disorders like diabetes, and affects mental health as well.

Sleep deficit accumulates over time, and if you experience sleeplessness several days each week, it will affect your work (impaired concentration, slowed reaction time, poor performance); relationships (impatience, crankiness, irritable behavior); and safety (driving and workplace accidents).

Sleep Deprivation Signals

By now, you're probably in tune with the signs of sleep deprivation. Here are some of them at a glance:

- Impaired memory or shortened attention span

- Loss of temper and irritability

- Dozing off while driving a car or in a meeting

- Hitting the alarm clock snooze button repeatedly

- Feeling unmotivated or lacking energy to "get going"

The sleep cycle and "normal" sleep

Identifying a "normal" night's sleep can be a challenge. For Rob, 42, normal is snoring away the first hours of the night, and tossing and turning until daybreak. Maybe for you, taking hours to fall asleep is part of the routine. You've seen more infomercials than you care to admit and have watched endless reruns.

It's true that sleep is different for each of us. So what is normal anyway? For decades, scientists pondered that question. Sleep research has helped identify what sleep is and how it differs from other states of mind.

After examining records from all-night sleep recordings, researchers noticed a predictable sequence of patterns over the course of a night. Overnight studies (which record a variety of body functions during sleep, including electrical activity in the brain, eye movements, muscle activity, heart rate, breathing effort, air flow through the nose and mouth, and oxygen levels) uncovered the "duality of sleep" or the difference between rapid eye movement (REM) sleep and non-rapid eye movement (NREM) sleep.

REM sleep is a mentally active period in which dreaming and rapid eye movements occur (you can observe this state in a sleeping cat) and the skeletal muscles of the body assume a paralyzed state. During NREM sleep, heart rate and breathing slow, and blood pressure decreases, while the body may twitch a few times as one falls asleep. We dream during NREM sleep, too. NREM sleep is divided into four stages, increasing in depth until REM sleep appears. Overnight sleep observations demonstrate how sleep normally progresses across the night. (See chart on following page.)

Normal Adult Histogram

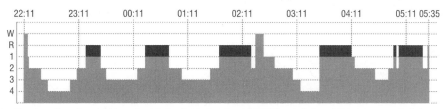

Note: Abundant Stage 3 and 4 (deep sleep) in the first half of the night. REM periods (in solid black) progressively increase as the night goes on; one awakening (bathroom break) a little after 2 a.m.

This histogram shows a night of sleep in a normal young adult. So, when Rob jolts out of sound sleep after only a few hours, chances are he completed only a portion of the full sleep cycle, leaving him deprived of true, sound sleep. Likewise, Ruth's constant waking indicates that her body probably never followed through the "normal" sleep cycle.

The histogram below depicts the restless night of a patient with insomnia.

Insomnia Histogram

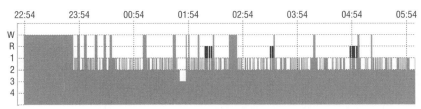

Note: Typical insomniac in sleep lab has a long sleep latency with frequent awakenings and little or no deep sleep (Stages 3 and 4) and REM. Similar pattern may be seen in people without insomnia who have difficulty sleeping due to the laboratory environment.

The sleep cycle

A sleep period begins with NREM sleep, which usually constitutes 75 to 80 percent of sleep time. NREM sleep is divided into four stages.

- **Stage 1:** 5 to 10 percent of sleep time.
- **Stage 2:** 30 to 50 percent of sleep time.

    Stages 1 and 2 are light sleep.

- **Stages 3 and 4:** 20 to 40 percent of sleep time.

    Stages 3 and 4 are deep sleep, or slow wave sleep (SWS).

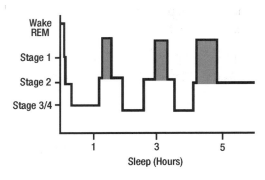

Shortly after the first SWS period, the body enters REM sleep, which constitutes 20 to 25 percent of sleep time. REM sleep is a mentally active period characterized by bursts of rapid eye movements. During this time, dreaming occurs and the brain is in fast-forward – so are blood pressure, heart rate, and other body functions when compared to SWS. Though the body is paralyzed during REM sleep, brain activity is intense. Scientists learned that subjects who are awakened during REM sleep remember their dreams, and that dreams vary in length depending on the REM sleep cycle. A complete sleep cycle generally takes ninety minutes. Adults have four to six sleep cycles during the night.

REM sleep is evidence that sleep is complex and not a halfway point to coma or death. The discovery of REM sleep in 1953 changed the way that researchers explained sleep. Understanding that the body is not completely "at rest," but instead recharging, further defines sleep's role in body and health restoration.

When Should I Talk to the Doctor?

One of the primary signals of a sleep disorder is whether the problem (insomnia or sleepiness) adversely affects daytime functioning. We often forget that sleep disorders also include problems with wakefulness – in other words, difficulty staying awake after sleeping all night.

Ask yourself the following questions:

- Do you regularly (at least a couple of times per week) have trouble falling asleep at night?

- Are you tired and lagging most days, despite a good night's sleep?

Sleep hygiene

Sleep hygiene (lifestyle and dietary habits that affect sleep behavior) is mostly a matter of common sense – avoiding caffeine late in the day, moderating alcohol intake, and creating an inviting environment for sleep (a dark, quiet room is best). Chapter 8 will address sleep hygiene more as it relates to insomnia.

But as you consider whether your disruptive sleep behavior is actually a sleep disorder and cause for medical attention, ask yourself these questions pertaining to your sleep hygiene:

- Do you go to bed at the same time every night?
- Do you use the bed for activities like watching television and reading?
- Is your bedroom conducive to sleep?
- Are your sleep patterns the same on weekdays and weekends?
- Are your waking times irregular?

A few words about drowsy driving

Don't underestimate the danger of getting behind the wheel after a sleepless night. Drowsy driving is as fatal as drunk driving. Nine out of ten North American police officers have stopped a driver who they believed was drunk but turned out to be drowsy, according to the 2004 American Automobile Association Foundation for Traffic Safety Internet survey. When sleep-deprived drivers get behind the wheel, their motor skills, alertness, and performance are impaired. Drowsiness plays into 100,000 police-reported crashes annually, according to the U.S. National Highway Traffic Safety Administration.

Sleep history

The sleep history is obtained during an interview with a physician. During this time, a physician will gather critical information necessary to diagnose a potential sleep disorder, tailor an overnight sleep study so it meets your specific needs, and designate an appropriate treatment program.

Some sleep centers ask patients to complete a questionnaire addressing sleep habits and complaints. This questionnaire is important, but not a surrogate for a one-on-one interview with a sleep specialist. This questionnaire provides you with an opportunity to list your primary problem and related behaviors that affect your ability to sleep soundly.

Starting with basic gender, height, and weight information, the sleep history expands into more detailed subjects, such as whether you work a second or third shift, your preferred sleeping position, and whether you take prescription or over-the-counter drugs to help you sleep.

You can expect to discuss the following topics with your physician during a sleep interview:

- Sleep habits

- Daytime sleepiness

- Nighttime behaviors

- Childhood sleep

A sleep interview is the first step toward a sleep disorder diagnosis. Oftentimes, sleep specialists use additional questionnaires to help paint a picture of your sleeping habits at night and alertness levels during the day. Depending on how you respond, your sleep patterns can be compared to normal ones.

The sleep interview is a one-on-one conversation between you and your doctor. Standardized questionnaires that ask you to consider your habits and activities can help the doctor determine whether testing in a sleep laboratory is necessary. Many times, the sleep interview provides a doctor with enough information to diagnose a sleep disorder and develop a treatment program.

The different sleep scales

Doctors discover sleep patterns by charting activity throughout a twenty-four-hour period. Your doctor may ask you to keep a sleep log or diary for a week or two, maybe more. Sleep logs can help your doctor identify problems such as insufficient sleep as a cause of daytime sleepiness or irregular sleep-wake cycles.

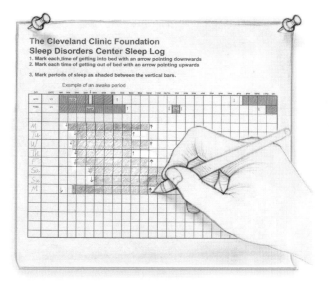

Sleep specialists use a variety of questionnaires designed to screen for different sleep, medical and psychiatric disorders. Some of the most commonly used questionnaires in sleep clinics are the following:

1. The Epworth Sleepiness Scale

This scale asks you to rate how likely you are to fall sleep in certain situations as opposed to just feeling tired. You should rate your sleepiness based on your recent lifestyle. Even if you have not participated in some of these activities lately, imagine how your body might respond.

The Epworth Sleepiness Scale questionnaire uses the following scale:
>   0 = would **never** doze
>   1 = **slight** chance of dozing
>   2 = **moderate** chance of dozing
>   3 = **high** chance of dozing

Situation	Chance of Dozing			
	never	slight	moderate	high
• Sitting and reading				
• Watching TV				
• Sitting inactive in a public place (e.g., a theater or meeting)				
• As a passenger in a car without a break				
• Lying down to rest in the afternoon when circumstances permit				
• Sitting and talking to someone				
• Sitting quietly after a lunch without alcohol				
• In a car while stopped for a few minutes in traffic				

The eight responses are tallied, producing a score from 0 to 24, with higher scores indicating more significant degrees of sleepiness. A score of 10 or greater is considered abnormal and signifies daytime sleepiness.

2. The Fatigue Severity Scale

This scale asks you to choose a number from 1 to 7 that indicates your level of agreement with each statement (1 = strongly agree; 7 = strongly disagree). It is a measure of the impact of fatigue on how a person functions.

1. My motivation is lower when I am fatigued.
2. Exercise brings on my fatigue.
3. I am easily fatigued.
4. Fatigue interferes with my physical conditioning.
5. Fatigue causes frequent problems for me.
6. My fatigue prevents sustained physical functioning.
7. Fatigue interferes with carrying out certain duties and responsibilities.
8. Fatigue is among my three most disabling symptoms.
9. Fatigue interferes with my work, family, or social life.

The nine responses are tallied with results ranging from 0 to 63. A score of 36 or higher is abnormal, indicating significant functional impairment due to fatigue.

3. Beck Depression Inventory

This questionnaire is commonly used to screen for depression, which often is present with sleep complaints. There are twenty-one categories of statements. Patients choose the one that best describes how they have been feeling the past week, including today. If several statements in the group apply equally well, they mark each one.

This test is scored from 0 to 63. Cutoffs used by the Massachusetts General Hospital and many sleep specialists are the following:

0-7: Normal

7-15: Mild

15-25: Moderate

25+: Severe

See Appendix 3 for the Beck Depression Inventory.

A to Zzzzs – Some Helpful Terms

Polysomnogram (PSG): An overnight study that takes place in a sleep lab.

Multiple Sleep Latency Test (MSLT): A daytime test consisting of a series of naps performed in a sleep laboratory after an overnight sleep study. The purpose is to evaluate the complaint of daytime sleepiness.

Good sleep hygiene: Habits that promote healthy sleep, such as maintaining regular bed/wake-up times, avoiding caffeine and alcohol before bed, and using your bed only for sleep.

Sleep latency: How long it takes a person to fall asleep. For example, if your sleep latency is five minutes, you fall asleep easily.

Sleep onset: When a person first falls asleep.

Sleep stages: The sleep cycle comprises four stages of sleep called non-rapid eye movement (NREM) plus rapid eye movement (REM) sleep. We progress through the cycle several times each night.

Chapter 3
Do You Need a Sleep Study?

> *A good laugh and a long sleep are the best cures*
> *in the doctor's book.*
>
> *– Irish proverb*

Most adults have had difficulty getting a good night's sleep or have experienced daytime sleepiness at some point in their lives. Environmental conditions and life changes that provoke periods of emotional distress – a death in the family, divorce – can trigger a temporary bout of insomnia. Sleep loss to make a deadline may lead to daytime sleepiness or poor performance on the job. This is normal, and the problem will resolve once a normal sleep pattern is reestablished.

But what should you do if a few nights of lost sleep multiply into weeks, months, or even years? What about when daytime sleepiness or fatigue occurs even after seemingly good nights of sleep? A sleep disorder can last a short period, or it can develop into a health-threatening illness that affects all aspects of your life.

Getting professional help

In order to determine whether your sleep complaint is cause for concern, your doctor will want to collect facts about your sleep-wake patterns and may request that you maintain a log that details time in bed, time asleep, nighttime behavior, and feelings of fatigue or sleepiness during the day. Of course, you won't know the answers to every question a physician asks you about your sleep habits. You might deny snoring until a bed partner complains. You might not realize that you stop breathing in your sleep; you only know that you wake frequently during the night and are tired most days.

If you report excessive daytime sleepiness, your physician will probably recommend an overnight sleep study. Excessive sleepiness almost always signifies a sleep disorder, although medical disorders and medications (including over-the-counter drugs) may contribute. Patients who experience daytime sleepiness might suffer from such common sleep disorders as insufficient sleep syndrome, sleep apnea, or narcolepsy.

And while patients who complain of insomnia generally benefit more from clinical treatment, sometimes an overnight sleep test can shed new light on their sleep habits. Some insomniacs have false impressions of exactly how many hours they spend sleeping each night. This is called sleep-state misperception, and it is common among those with psychophysiological insomnia and insomnia related to psychiatric disorders. A tailored overnight sleep study is another piece of the diagnostic puzzle.

The polysomnogram, a test conducted during an overnight stay in a sleep lab, is a critical tool in evaluating, diagnosing, and treating sleep disorders because it reveals information you probably don't know about your own sleep. Conducted during an eight-hour period, it provides a detailed picture of your sleep-wake patterns over the course of one night. (The test also can take place during the day if a person works third shift or has other special circumstances.)

The polysomnogram

During the polysomnogram, a technologist monitors the following functions:

- **EEG:** An electroencephalogram records brain-wave activity, which indicates whether a person is awake or asleep and identifies the various stages of sleep (NREM stages 1 through 4 and REM). Four to six (sometimes more) sensors, also known as electrodes, are placed at precise locations on the head.

- **EOG:** Electro-oculography refers to the recording of eye movements. Slow eye movements occur during drowsiness, and rapid eye movements take place during REM sleep and wakefulness. Electrodes are attached to the skin at the outside corner of each eye.

- **EMG:** In electromyography, electrodes are placed over muscles to record movements and muscle tone. In overnight sleep studies, EMG electrodes are placed on the chin to detect changes in muscle tone. This helps determine sleep stages. During REM sleep, for example, the tone of skeletal muscles is very low as the body completely relaxes and, in fact, is paralyzed. (At the same time, eye movement speeds up, as detected by the EOG.) EMG electrodes are also placed over specified muscles in the arms and legs, in particular over the shins, to measure periodic and random leg movements, which can interfere with sleep quality.

- **EKG:** An electrocardiogram is recorded during overnight sleep tests through sensors placed on the chest. These measure heart rate and rhythm during sleep and wakefulness. When a patient lacks oxygen, heart rate can slow down, speed up, or fall into an abnormal rhythm. (This applies to sleep apnea sufferers, who stop breathing – or have "apneas" – for ten seconds or longer at a time.)

- **Respiration:** Airflow from the nose and mouth must be recorded to identify periods of complete or partial interruptions in breathing during sleep. A sensor is placed in or near the nostril and outside the mouth. In some cases, an additional cannula, or slender tube, is positioned near the nose to measure the amount of carbon dioxide in exhaled air. Two belts placed around the chest and abdomen measure breathing effort during sleep.

- **Oxygen Saturation:** By measuring the oxygen level, the technologist can determine whether apneic events are producing significant drops in oxygen during sleep. To do this, a pulse oximeter probe is placed over the fingertip or ear lobe.

- **Body Position:** The technologist records unusual body movement and sleep position by observing a live video of patients while they sleep. Video usage is becoming mainstream in sleep laboratories. Before the study begins, the technologist will indicate whether patients will be recorded and often obtain a consent in writing.

- **Snoring:** A snore microphone is taped to the lateral neck area.

Preparing for a sleep study

The overnight sleep study should be tailored to fit your needs. To ensure that it will address your sleep concerns, your primary physician will be required to provide the sleep center with a recent medical history and physical examination prior to the test, as well as some details about the reason the test has been ordered (i.e., snoring, daytime sleepiness). Many centers will ask you to maintain a log of your sleep and wake times, including naps, for one to two weeks before testing. A sleep log not only provides insight to the technologist or physician who performs and reads (or "scores") your polysomnogram, it also can help you understand your problem better.

Additionally, patients often are requested to fill out questionnaires, like the Epworth Sleepiness Scale, prior to an overnight study. You might receive these questions in advance or be asked to answer them after you check into the sleep lab for your test. This information is a critical component of the overnight study, preparing sleep specialists with your sleep history information so they can better interpret the results.

Your sleep history information will cover:

- Snoring

- Witnessed apneas

- Choking or gasping during sleep

- Excessive daytime sleepiness

- Daytime fatigue

- Impaired concentration

- Difficulty falling sleep because of uncomfortable legs

- Recurrent awakenings from sleep

- Unusual night behavior

- Excessive movements during sleep

- Medical history

- Past surgeries

- Medications, alcohol, and recreational drug use

- Weight change over time

- History of childhood sleep problems

- Family history of sleep disorders

What to expect at the sleep lab

If sleeping soundly at home is a rarity, the thought of catching some zzzs in an unfamiliar place may seem impossible, especially if you know you'll be recorded and observed during the process. However, most patients who check into a sleep lab for an overnight study sleep better than they expect. They are exhausted in the first place.

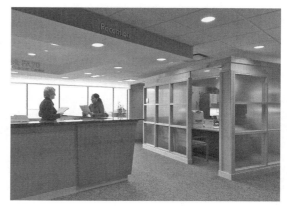

Also, sleep labs are designed to be comfortable. Your room will likely resemble a hotel suite. Sleep labs typically are outpatient facilities, which don't have the clinical feel of a hospital setting. Of course, medical elements aren't removed from the equation. The nightstand in your sleep lab room might contain controllers and devices necessary to conduct the polysomnogram.

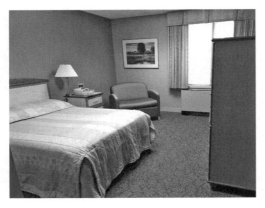

Because of a burgeoning demand for overnight sleep studies, many medical centers have expanded their sleep labs to locations outside the medical center's campus, like hotels in nearby communities. The Cleveland Clinic is one such health system; its Sleep Disorders Center opened branches in Courtyard Marriott hotels. This has been a popular choice for patients.

Regardless of whether your sleep lab appointment is in the hospital, an outpatient clinic, or an equipped hotel setting, you will be greeted and introduced to the process when you check in. You will arrive for your study in the evening, usually a couple of hours before your normal bedtime. (Check with the sleep center for specifics.) You will be shown to your room and given time to settle in, change into bedclothes, and relax for a while. A technologist will then hook you up for the study, which can take up to an hour or longer, depending on the nature of your test. He or she will place electrodes and sensors on your head, chin, and legs, and sensors around your nose, mouth, chest, and abdomen. These electrodes are connected to wires, which will be gathered into a ponytail behind your head so you can roll over and change positions as you sleep.

Ask questions while these devices are being applied. The technologist can ease concerns about the process and explain why each measurement device is important for learning about your sleep patterns. Also, be sure to mention any morning commitments. That way, you can arrange an appropriate wake-up call. Tests usually last until 6 or 6:30 a.m., and some patients are required to stay the entire next day for daytime testing. Because most sleep centers are in outpatient settings manned by technologists (not nurses), expect to bring and take your own medications during your stay. Notify the sleep center in advance if you or a loved one has special needs.

Pre-testing do's and don'ts

Following these guidelines will ensure that your test is accurate and the best possible example of "normal" sleep for you:

- Avoid taking a nap on the day of the study.

- Avoid alcohol, caffeine, sedatives, and stimulants for twenty-four hours before the study, unless otherwise specified by your doctor. In some cases, patients using stimulants are advised to continue their usual medications.

- Eat your regular evening meal before you arrive at the sleep lab.

- On the day of the study, make sure your hair is free of oil, hair spray, and other products.

- Bring your medications and plan to take them as you normally would, unless a physician instructs otherwise.

- Bring sleepwear that is comfortable (PJs are better than nightgowns), but avoid silk.

- Bring the completed sleep questionnaires if paperwork was given to you before the study.

- If you are using positive airway pressure therapy at home, bring your mask.

- Pack an overnight bag with toiletries, bedclothes, and your own pillow if you prefer.

Minors and adults with special needs are typically required to have a guardian or caregiver present during the study. Many labs have accommodations, such as a pullout sofa, where a family member can stay the night.

Behind the scenes

While patients sleep, the technologists stay busy. In the "control room," they watch video screens and log body position and unusual movements. They listen for snoring and abrupt breathing noises, and observe brain, eye, and breathing activity on a computer screen (thus the reason for the electrodes). They take notes as they notice behavior in various sleep stages. For example, if they detect leg movement (common with periodic limb movement syndrome in early sleep stages), they note this on a sleep chart.

If breathing problems are observed, a technologist might wake you up and ask you to try a continuous positive airway pressure device. This sits on the night-stand and includes a mask that fits around your nose and/or mouth. The machine forces air into the mask and into your airway, keeping it open so you can breathe and sleep better. It is not necessary for all patients, but depends on the severity of the breathing difficulty.

When you wake up, the technologist stops the recording. You may be asked to fill out a questionnaire that will include such questions as:

1) How long did it take you to fall asleep last night?

2) How does this compare with the length of time it usually takes you to fall asleep?

3) How long do you feel you slept last night?

4) How many times did you wake up last night?

After the study is complete, the technologist "scores" the polysomnogram. One night's recordings can consume 1,000 to 1,500 feet of paper. (This is one reason most laboratories now record data using computer systems instead of paper machines.) It will take the technologist several hours to analyze this information and compile it into a sleep report.

A sleep report will include the following:

Time in Bed: Time from lights out to lights on, in minutes.

Total Sleep Time: Total time spent in stages 1 through 4 and REM, in minutes.

Sleep Latency: Time from lights out to the first appearance of sleep, in minutes.

REM Latency: Time from sleep onset to the first appearance of REM, in minutes.

Sleep Efficiency: Time in bed spent in sleep, expressed as a percentage.

Sleep Stage Percentage: Time spent in each sleep stage divided by the total sleep time, expressed as a percentage.

Apnea/Hypopnea Indices: Number of apneic or hypopneic events per sleep hour. (Apnea is total obstruction of the airway; hypopnea is partial obstruction in breathing. Read more in Chapter 5.)

Arousal Index: Number of times per sleep hour an arousal from sleep occurs.

Oxygen Data: Number of times a patient has a significant reduction in oxygen, and the amount of sleep time spent with subnormal oxygen levels (expressed as a percentage).

PLMI Data: Number of periodic limb movements per sleep hour. (Less than five per hour is normal for people under the age of 60. The cutoff is higher for mature adults, as PLMs increase with age.)

PLMAI Data: Number of periodic limb movements per sleep hour that cause arousals. Many people have PLMs, but physicians pay close attention when these movements trigger an arousal from sleep.

Once a technologist scores the study, a sleep specialist reviews it and prepares a report for your physician. This is based on the recording in the lab and your sleep history. More than 2,000 variables are collected during an overnight sleep study, and the digitized programs in sleep recording systems crunch all of these numbers. A doctor can find out whether you snore while you sleep on your back or your right side. This may seem an insignificant detail, but it is important to know whether body position caused an apneic episode or whether disruptions in breathing occurred during a certain sleep stage. Tailored sleep study reports shed light on the intricacies of how we sleep.

After an overnight sleep study, your doctor may refer you for a consultation with a sleep specialist to discuss the results, diagnosis, and treatment, as well as sleep hygiene and lifestyle changes critical to therapy.

First-night effect

The unusual environment of a sleep lab affects sleep patterns. Patients may display highly abnormal sleep because they cannot get comfortable in the new setting. This is called first-night effect. In some cases, a physician may request that a patient return to the clinic for a second study.

Reading the lines

Polysomnograms are like sleep maps: The squiggly, wavy, and sometimes flat lines that recordings produce tell physicians whether a patient displays symptoms of a sleep disorder. These studies are critical to correct diagnosis and treatment.

But what do the lines mean?

Below is an EEG (brain wave) tracing of a patient who is awake. You will notice the lines are random and fast.

Wake

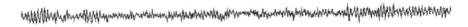

Below, you will notice the slower waves of a patient who is drowsy.

Stage 1

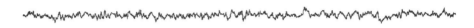

This recording displays theta waves of stage 1 sleep. These waves are repetitive and look like small, jagged mountains. They are still relatively low voltage. During this stage, the eyes may rove back and forth as seen on an EOG tracing.

In the tracing below, you will notice a "sleep spindle" and "K complex" inherent in stage 2 sleep.

Stage 2   K complex/sleep spindle

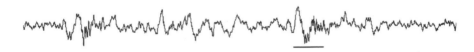

Stages 3 and 4 are characterized by high-voltage, slow delta waves. During normal sleep, you will spend most of the night in stages 2 through 4.

Stages 3 and 4/Slow Wave Sleep

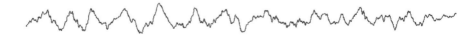

REM sleep occurs approximately ninety minutes from sleep onset and can happen three or more times a night. (It can occur less often if a patient displays problems transitioning from one sleep stage to the next.) These low voltage waves are random and fast with sawtooth waves.

REM Sleep

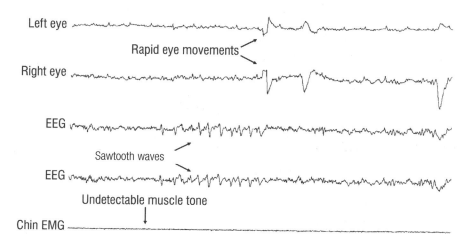

The figure on page 14 shows how a person progresses through normal sleep.

In cases of sleep apnea, video recordings are especially helpful because technologists can observe a patient's sleep position. For some patients, sleep apnea occurs only when they're sleeping on their backs. (This is common, as the position causes the tongue to flop backward, blocking the upper airway as shown in the figure below.) The technologist will attempt to record sleep in both positions (side and back, or supine) and in the patient's usual sleep position (which might include sitting in a recliner). This allows the technologist to observe whether the patient displays symptoms of sleep apnea in that position.

Daytime sleep testing – the MSLT

After the polysomnogram, your physician might request that you stay at the sleep lab for a multiple sleep latency test or MSLT. This is a series of nap trials that take place approximately two hours after waking from the overnight sleep study. The MSLT is the gold-standard test used in the evaluation of daytime sleepiness. The test consists of five nap trials, performed at two-hour intervals, the day after an adequate night's sleep. This test indicates whether a patient has excessive daytime sleepiness and measures its severity. It is an important test for patients suspected of having narcolepsy, a disorder marked by uncontrollable sudden sleep attacks during active situations such as eating, talking, and even driving.

Take Elizabeth, who stayed the morning after her overnight sleep study for an MSLT. She presented with symptoms of narcolepsy, but her physician ordered a polysomnogram to get a better picture of how she spends her nights. The MSLT was critical to diagnosing her sleep disorder because the physician discovered how very little time it took Elizabeth to fall asleep the morning after the sleep study even after sleeping well at night.

When the technologist entered her room to prepare her for the first nap trial, she was sound asleep seconds after he turned off the light. In the control room, the technologist noticed that Elizabeth entered REM – abnormal behavior for a "nap." Elizabeth was awakened and did not realize how soundly she had slept. Nearly two hours later, it was time for the second nap trial. She fell asleep just as quickly.

The MSLT is based on the assumption that sleep is critical to function. When a patient is sleep-deprived or has a disorder in which wakefulness is impaired, the body will shut down. Electrodes placed on the head measuring brain waves and eye movements indicate how deeply a patient sleeps during nap trials. Patients who fall asleep in five minutes or less display signs of severe, excessive daytime sleepiness. (Normally rested individuals generally do not fall asleep in less than ten minutes in this situation.)

Daytime testing preparation

If you stay at the sleep lab for the MSLT, a technologist will wake you up after your night study and remove the respiratory, oxygen, and leg sensors. Only brain activity, eye movements, and muscle tone over the chin are measured during the MSLT, and these recordings are captured using the same electrodes applied the night before.

Most sleep laboratories will provide a light breakfast before the test begins. No sooner than ninety minutes after you wake up, the technologist will return to the room to prepare you for your first nap. Lights will be turned out and other distractions removed. Your sleep patterns are monitored during this time. This test lasts most of the day, so call the sleep lab in advance to find out detailed information about breakfast, lunch, and the approximate time the study will end. During the day, you can take prescribed medications as usual, unless otherwise instructed by a physician.

You will not be permitted to consume stimulants, alcohol, or caffeine unless

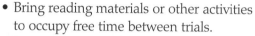

otherwise directed by your physician. (Yes, this includes your morning coffee!)

- Bring reading materials or other activities to occupy free time between trials.
- Wear comfortable clothing.
- Avoid naps, smoking, or physical exertion prior to the test and in between nap trials.

The amount you sleep during these nap trials helps physicians understand complaints of daytime sleepiness, fatigue, and disrupted sleep at night. The MSLT uncovers information critical to making an accurate sleep disorder diagnosis and is important to designing a treatment plan.

Chapter 4

Sleep Diagnosis & the International Classification of Sleep Disorders

Sleeping is no mean art:
for its sake one must stay awake all day.
— *Nietzsche*

Considering what is known about normal sleep and how the body should transition from one sleep stage to the next, physicians can distinguish sleep disruptions that originate within the body from those initiated by outside influences. An overnight sleep study, questionnaires, and sleep logs are tools to help physicians diagnose sleep disorders. *The International Classification of Sleep Disorders* (2nd ed.) was produced by the American Academy of Sleep Medicine in 2005. The manual describes the currently recognized sleep disorders based on available medical evidence. It serves as a sleep disorders bible for specialists.

There are more than eighty distinct sleep disorders, which fall under eight main categories:

1. Insomnias

2. Sleep-Related Breathing Disorders

3. Hypersomnias of Central Origin Not Due to a Circadian Rhythm Sleep Disorder, Sleep-Related Breathing Disorder, or Other Cause of Disturbed Nocturnal Sleep

4. Circadian Rhythm Sleep Disorders

5. Parasomnias

6. Sleep-Related Movement Disorders

7. Isolated Symptoms, Apparently Normal Variants, and Unresolved Issues

8. Other Sleep Disorders

Following is a list of sleep disorders, arranged by category. This book addresses seven of them through patient case studies: Obstructive Sleep Apnea, Narcolepsy, Restless Legs Syndrome, Psychophysiological Insomnia, Delayed Phase Sleep Disorder, Sleep Terrors/SleepWalking, and REM Behavior Disorder.

Additionally, it addresses sleep disorders in the same "families" as these cases.

Insomnia

Adjustment Insomnia (Acute Insomnia)
Psychophysiological Insomnia
Paradoxical Insomnia
Idiopathic Insomnia
Insomnia Due to Mental Disorder
Inadequate Sleep Hygiene
Behavioral Insomnia of Childhood
Insomnia Due to Drug or Substance
Insomnia Due to Medical Condition
Insomnia Not Due to Substance or Known Physiological Condition, Unspecified
Physiological (Organic) Insomnia, Unspecified

Sleep-Related Breathing Disorders

Central Sleep Apnea Syndromes
    Primary Central Sleep Apnea
    Central Sleep Apnea Due to Cheyne-Stokes Breathing Pattern
    Central Sleep Apnea Due to High-Altitude Periodic Breathing
    Central Sleep Apnea Due to Medical Condition Not Cheyne-Stokes
    Central Sleep Apnea Due to Drug or Substance
    Primary Sleep Apnea of Infants
    (Formerly Primary Sleep Apnea of Newborns)
Obstructive Sleep Apnea Syndromes
    Obstructive Sleep Apnea, Adult
    Obstructive Sleep Apnea, Pediatric
Sleep-Related Hypoventilation/Hypoxemic Syndromes
    Sleep-Related Nonobstructive Alveolar Hypoventilation, Idiopathic
    Congenital Central Alveolar Hypoventilation Syndrome
Sleep-Related Hypoventilation/Hypoxemia Due to Medical Condition
    Sleep-Related Hypoventilation/Hypoxemia Due to Pulmonary
      Parenchymal or Vascular Pathology
    Sleep-Related Hypoventilation/Hypoxemia Due to Lower Airway
      Obstruction
    Sleep-Related Hypoventilation/Hypoxemia Due to Neuromuscular and
      Chest Wall Disorders
Other Sleep-Related Breathing Disorder
    Sleep Apnea/Sleep-Related Breathing Disorder, Unspecified

Hypersomnias of Central Origin Not Due to a Circadian Rhythm Sleep Disorder, Sleep-Related Breathing Disorder, or Other Cause of Disturbed Nocturnal Sleep

Narcolepsy with Cataplexy
Narcolepsy without Cataplexy
Narcolepsy Due to Medical Condition
Narcolepsy, Unspecified
Recurrent Hypersomnia
    Kleine-Levin Syndrome
    Menstrual-Related Hypersomnia
Idiopathic Hypersomnia with Long Sleep Time
Idiopathic Hypersomnia without Long Sleep Time
Behaviorally Induced Insufficient Sleep Syndrome
Hypersomnia Due to Medical Condition
Hypersomnia Due to Drug or Substance
Hypersomnia Not Due to Substance or Known Physiological Condition
Physiological Hypersomnia, Unspecified

Circadian Rhythm Sleep Disorders

Circadian Rhythm Sleep Disorder, Delayed Sleep Phase Disorder
Circadian Rhythm Sleep Disorder, Advanced Sleep Phase Disorder
Circadian Rhythm Sleep Disorder, Irregular Sleep-Wake Rhythm
Circadian Rhythm Sleep Disorder, Free-Running Type
Circadian Rhythm Sleep Disorder, Jet Lag Disorder
Circadian Rhythm Sleep Disorder, Shift Work Disorder
Circadian Rhythm Sleep Disorder Due to Medical Condition
Other Circadian Rhythm Sleep Disorder
Other Circadian Rhythm Sleep Disorder Due to Drug or Substance

Parasomnias

Disorders of Arousal (from NREM Sleep)
    Confusional Arousals
    Sleepwalking
    Sleep Terrors
Parasomnias Usually Associated with REM Sleep
    REM Behavior Disorder
    Recurrent Isolated Sleep Paralysis
    Nightmare Disorder

Other Parasomnias

    Sleep-Related Dissociative Disorders
    Sleep Enuresis
    Sleep-Related Groaning
    Exploding Head Syndrome
    Sleep-Related Hallucinations
    Sleep-Related Eating Disorder
    Parasomnia, Unspecified
    Parasomnia Due to Drug or Substance
    Parasomnia Due to Medical Condition

Sleep-Related Movement Disorders

Restless Legs Syndrome
Periodic Limb Movement Disorder
Sleep-Related Leg Cramps
Sleep-Related Bruxism
Sleep-Related Rhythmic Movement Disorder
Sleep-Related Movement Disorder, Unspecified
Sleep-Related Movement Disorder Due to Drug or Substance
Sleep-Related Movement Disorder Due to Medical Condition

Isolated Symptoms, Apparently Normal Variants and Unresolved Issues

Long Sleeper
Short Sleeper
Snoring
Sleeptalking
Sleep Starts (Hypnic Jerks)
Benign Sleep Myoclonus of Infancy
Hypnagogic Foot Tremor and Alternating Leg Muscle Activation
    During Sleep
Propriospinal Myoclonus at Sleep Onset
Excessive Fragmentary Myoclonus

Other Sleep Disorders

Other Physiological (Organic) Sleep Disorder
Other Sleep Disorder Not Due to Substance or Known
    Physiological Condition
Environmental Sleep Disorder

Sleep Disorders Associated with Other Conditions

Beyond this list are sleep disorders associated with psychiatric, behavioral, and physical conditions. Mood disorders, anxiety, depression, schizophrenia, and other psychotic and personality disorders will contribute to a person's inability to sleep. A physician must determine whether the individual does, in fact, present with a primary sleep disorder or whether the sleep problems are due to psychiatric or behavioral disorders.

Medical conditions that disrupt sleep include sleep-related epilepsy, headaches, gastroesophageal reflux, and chest pains and pulmonary disorders such as COPD. Remember, sleep affects our whole health – and psychological and physical conditions certainly play into our ability to get a good night's sleep.

Chapter 5

Obstructive Sleep Apnea

Laugh and the world laughs with you;
snore and you sleep alone.

– Anthony Burgess

Obstructive sleep apnea *is characterized by repetitive episodes of complete (apnea) or partial (hypopnea) upper airway obstruction during sleep. Often the disorder's first signs are snoring, gasping for breath during sleep, and excessive daytime sleepiness.*

Dan, 43, drove to work early one morning, groggy as usual, his "go" cup filled with his third cup of coffee propped on the dashboard. He lapsed into a daze, staring blankly at the road before him, ticks of yellow road stripe blurring by his sideview mirror. His speed gradually slowed to five miles less than the limit while his car crept closer to the berm.

Dan jolted awake when his head bobbed and he realized with a gasp that he had almost driven his car into the highway ditch. He exhaled anxiously. He sleeps about eight hours each night but never wakes up feeling refreshed. The coffee certainly didn't help that morning – it never does.

Why am I so tired every day? He considered the last time he was not exhausted in the morning. That was four years ago.

His wife, Karen, hasn't been too cheery in the morning, either. She is used to his daily naps and lazy weekends, but his loud snoring tests her patience. She has developed a few night karate moves designed to stop his snarking. She elbows him in the gut and rolls him from his preferred supine sleeping position to his side. Usually, she resorts to pulling the covers over her head to muffle the sound. Dan's hacking and wheezing remind her of a squawking duck. For his part, Dan is oblivious to the problem until she complains in the morning. Some nights she retreats to the living-room sofa.

Dan is a sturdy man with a thick neck and large frame. His body mass index is 38 (normal is 18.5 to 24.9), and his family doctor warned him to watch his fast-food habit.

Three years ago, Dan was diagnosed with obstructive sleep apnea and treated with continuous positive airway pressure (CPAP), by a machine that delivers air into the nose and/or mouth through a mask. Dan wore the mask regularly for a year, but he didn't notice any benefit. He stopped using it until recently. Karen asked him to ease back into CPAP therapy, hoping it would reduce his labored breathing. It hasn't. They both know that Dan needs to seek treatment again.

Dan's sleep assessment

Sleep snapshot

Dan, an electrician, averages eight hours of sleep each night. More sleep generally does not make him feel more refreshed during the day. Typically he dozes off and on beginning at 6 p.m., shortly after dinner, while lounging in front of the television. Karen wakes him up to go to bed a few hours later.

He usually wakes up two times during the night, for the following reasons: snoring, reflux symptoms, a leg or arm jerk, or because he needs to use the bathroom. But Karen suspects he wakes up much more as she observes him tossing and turning, his body jolting and snoring throughout the night. He never has a problem falling back asleep after one of these episodes.

Dan wakes up every morning at 5 and arrives at work no later than 7:30, often with a headache. He generally finishes his last electrical job at 3:30 p.m. But last year during his annual performance evaluation, his supervisor noted that Dan was "losing his edge" and not quite as efficient as he had been in the past. Dan recalls shocking himself when he started to nod off in the middle of an electrical wiring job.

Excessive daytime sleepiness

Despite the hours Dan clocks in bed each night, he rarely feels rested when he wakes in the morning. He usually sneaks in two catnaps during his breaks at work. On Saturdays, he sometimes picks up overtime shifts, but if he has free time and is not scheduled to work, Dan will sleep the whole weekend.

Dan has lived with excessive daytime sleepiness for more than ten years, and like many patients who report this condition, he has grown accustomed to fatigue and learned to compensate or write it off as "no big deal." But when a wake-up call occurs in an automobile, sleepiness is a concern that deserves medical attention. Though Dan has never been issued a moving violation, he's come close to having an accident several times.

Medical history

After his overnight sleep study three years ago, Dan was diagnosed with obstructive sleep apnea (OSA) and treated with CPAP. He says this therapy has not helped him. His new physician could not locate prior evaluations or polysomnogram results.

Sleep-disordered breathing

Dan has never had nose or throat surgery and recalls no history of facial trauma. But his snoring has worsened in the last six years, and he's packed on more than thirty pounds, too. His snoring is especially bad when he falls asleep on his back. Dan says he sometimes stops breathing or gasps for air during sleep.

Most of the time, snoring has no serious side effects other than being an annoyance. Snoring is the sound that tissues in the nose and throat area make when the airway is not completely open. It is often the first indication of obstructive sleep apnea, and the physician immediately linked Dan's habit to his previous OSA diagnosis.

Physical examination

Dan shows no sign of overbite or enlarged tonsils – both indications that potentially point to OSA. His nasal airway is adequate, but the physician noticed that his mouth is characterized by a very low-lying soft palate. He has excessive tissue on his lateral pharyngeal wall, or pharynx area. Dan's neck circumference measures 18 inches, and patients with larger-sized collars are more susceptible to OSA (additional tissue can crowd the upper airway). His heart rate, blood pressure, and respiratory rate (the number of breaths per minute) are normal.

The physician was most concerned about Dan's neck size and upper airway structure, two physical traits typical of patients with OSA.

The diagnosis

The physician referred Dan to the sleep laboratory where another overnight sleep study confirmed the previous diagnosis of OSA. During the study, Dan stopped breathing forty-two times per hour (that's an apnea-hypopnea index of 42); he spent about 25 percent of his sleep time with subnormal oxygen levels. The physician ordered an urgent polysomnogram with CPAP fitting. His home CPAP machine hadn't been checked or adjusted since he'd initially received it. If Dan's daytime sleepiness did not improve with this treatment, he would require further evaluation.

The physician asked Dan to discuss medical leave with his employer. She ordered no driving, operating heavy machinery or dangerous equipment, and no heights until his daytime sleepiness improved.

Further, the physician discussed treatment options with Dan, including general measures like avoiding alcohol before bed, losing weight, not sleeping on his back, and having surgery to correct physical obstructions in the airway passage.

All about obstructive sleep apnea

How do you know you have it?

Obstructive sleep apnea is one of the most common sleep disorders, with nearly 25 percent of men and 10 percent of women suffering from some degree of apnea. Often, bed partners are the first to discover early signs of OSA. Habitual snoring usually escalates in intensity before a patient is diagnosed with OSA. Many of those affected have no sleep complaints and feel refreshed when they wake up in the morning.

Though up to 30 percent of adults snore, those who present with OSA exhibit a loud, disruptive snoring pattern. Loud snores are followed by silence when a patient stops breathing, followed by a gasp for air – snore, silence, gasp. An OSA patient will repeat this cycle throughout the night with "apneic episodes," or periods when breathing stops and restarts.

Just as OSA patients generally do not realize the extent of their snoring, they also tend to overlook daytime sleepiness. As sleep deprivation becomes a cultural norm, exhausted individuals tend to downplay sleepiness, even when physicians question their level of alertness during the day.

Besides the familiar sound of OSA, other symptoms point to an OSA diagnosis. These include:

- Sudden awakenings following apneic episodes with a sensation of gasping, choking, or holding breath
- Daytime sleepiness, sleep attacks that are unintentional sleep episodes, unrefreshing sleep, fatigue, and rarely, insomnia
- Night sweats
- Morning dry mouth or sore throat from excessive snoring and respiratory stress
- Intellectual impairment, such as trouble concentrating, forgetfulness, or irritability

- Impotence

- Morning headaches

Certain physical traits and clinical features are highly characteristic of OSA. These include:

- Large neck circumference

- History of habitual snoring

- High body mass index, or excessive weight

- Structurally abnormal or crowded airway passages, including a number of physical blockages such as nasal obstruction, a low-hanging soft palate, a large uvula, or enlarged tonsils

- Hypertension (high blood pressure)

Symptoms in children are more subtle, but physicians commonly notice enlarged tonsils and adenoids. Surgery to remove tonsils is often helpful for children with OSA.

Another sign of OSA in children is sluggishness and poor performance in school. Daytime sleepiness often is misinterpreted as laziness in the classroom.

Following are other signs that a child might have OSA:

- Daytime mouth breathing and swallowing difficulty

- Inward movement of the rib cage when breathing in

- Unusual sleeping positions (such as sleeping on hands and knees or with the neck hyperextended)

- Agitated arousals

- Excessive sweating at night

- "Adenoidal face": dull expression, a bloated look, and swollen eyes

- Excessive daytime sleepiness

- Developmental delay, learning difficulties, decreased school performance, and behavioral disorders. *(There is a link between children with attention deficit disorder or attention deficit-hyperactivity disorder and OSA; up to 25 percent of children with ADD or ADHD might have OSA.)*

- Morning headaches

- Growth delay

- Frequent bed-wetting

Who is susceptible?

The portrait of a typical OSA patient looks a lot like Dan: a middle-aged, over-weight male with a large neck, longtime snoring habit, and a tendency to lag during the day. But this is not the only demographic suffering from OSA.

An estimated 3 million men and 1.5 million women in the United States show symptoms of OSA. And despite the 2:1 ratio of men to women who present with the disorder, the gender gap closes in later years when women are more susceptible due to hormonal changes. OSA, defined as at least five episodes of apnea or hypopnea per hour of sleep and excessive daytime sleepiness, affects 4 percent of men and 2 percent of women. When using the definition of five episodes of apnea (total obstruction of airway) or hypopnea (partial obstruction of airway) per sleep hour, 24 percent of men and 9 percent of women meet the criteria. As both men and women age, OSA symptoms are more prevalent, and all overweight individuals are at risk.

Additionally, more physicians are diagnosing patients with OSA, recognizing the disorder's morbidity in association with other serious medical problems, such as cardiovascular disease, hypertension, and stroke. Many of these problems also are linked to obesity. Most patients who have OSA are overweight and display weight gain prior to diagnosis.

What causes obstructive sleep apnea?

Sleep can be a potentially dangerous time for a person with OSA. During sleep, the muscles relax; this includes those in the throat. While partial collapse of air-way muscles causes snoring, complete collapse is an "apnea" or respiratory stop. Apnea comes from the Greek word meaning "without wind." In OSA patients, those muscles relax, narrow the breathing passages, and eventually collapse. This blockage causes apneic episodes – the snore, silence, gasp pattern familiar to bed partners of OSA sleepers.

Structural factors also inhibit the airway passage. Features such as an abnormally small jaw, large tongue, overbite, enlarged tonsils, or tissue that blocks the airway entrance contribute to OSA. A large neck circumference and extra tissue in the throat region, combined with a cramped airway, become a recipe for labored breathing during sleep. OSA in children is often due to congenital narrowing of the upper airway.

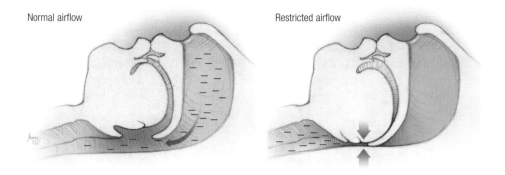

Normal airflow

Restricted airflow

Occasional apneas are normal, particularly in mature adults. But when apneas are repetitive and cause arousals, drops in a person's oxygen level, or changes in heart rate, they can contribute to more serious health problems.

The polysomnogram

During an overnight sleep study, a patient's nasal and oral airflow are monitored through sensors placed in or near nostrils and around the mouth. Two belts around the abdomen and rib cage measure breathing effort and are used to differentiate OSA from a rarer condition known as central sleep apnea. An oximeter probe placed on the fingertip provides a measure of oxygen levels, a surrogate for the level of oxygen in the blood. Many times, apneas cause repetitive drops in oxygen that deprive the brain and heart of this vital nutrient. A snore microphone is taped on the side of the neck to measure the intensity of snoring and correlate it with breathing patterns.

Obstructive Apnea

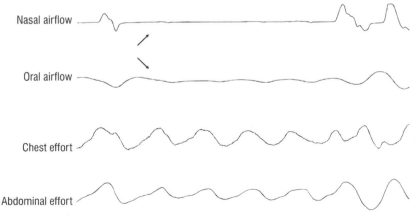

Nasal airflow

Oral airflow

Chest effort

Abdominal effort

Arrows indicate absent airflow through nose and mouth while breathing effort is preserved from the chest and abdominal muscles.

During an apneic episode, airflow through the nose and mouth stops, often causing an arousal and/or a change in heart rate. The heart typically will slow down (bradycardia) during the apnea and speed up (tachycardia) at the time of arousal. This is called a bradytachy response. The arousal is a reset button of sorts. After waking momentarily, patients catch their breath and fall back asleep. Most of the time, patients do not recognize these arousals. For example, Dan said he woke up only two times during the night. But his polysomnogram indicated that he was aroused from apneic episodes twenty-two times each hour.

Technologists look for breathing stops (apneic episodes) and episodes of significant breathing reduction (hypopneic episodes) that exceed ten seconds; most episodes last from twenty to forty seconds up to sixty to ninety seconds, though respiratory stops of this duration are rare. Episodes generally occur during NREM sleep stages 1 and 2, and they are more prevalent during REM. (Some patients experience these events only during REM sleep.)

How to get a good night's sleep

Treatment of OSA depends on severity. A physician might suggest general measures (such as abstaining from alcohol before bed, altering sleep position, losing weight) and/or therapeutic treatment. The latter includes positive airway pressure (PAP) therapy, oral appliances that help open the airway, or surgery to correct physical abnormalities of the upper airway that prevent normal nocturnal breathing. More often today, bariatric surgery is being considered for morbidly obese patients. Stimulants are used to treat residual daytime sleepiness in some cases.

No one formula works for every patient, and often a physician will employ a combination of these approaches to combat OSA. The key is to discuss treatment goals with the physician. Patients whose chief complaint is severe daytime sleepiness are not prime candidates for upper airway surgery, which will usually cure snoring but may not make them feel more awake during the day. Some patients adjust well to PAP therapy, while others cannot tolerate the machine. This is why education and a thorough assessment are critical precursors to any treatment plan.

General measures

- Weight loss: Weight gain can result in an excess of tissue in the neck region, which contributes to airway collapse. Even moderate weight loss can improve breathing during sleep.

- Avoiding alcohol and central nervous system depressants before bed: These agents relax muscle tone, including those in nasal and throat passages.

- Sleeping position: Some patients exhibit OSA only when they sleep on their backs. Tissue is more likely to "fall back" into the throat and prevent normal breathing. A side sleeping position is known to reduce apneic episodes. (Sleeping in a tight-fitting shirt with a tennis ball lodged in the back will prevent OSA patients from sleeping on their backs; so will a pillow or maternity wedge positioned at the back.)

- Nasal congestion: Those with sinus problems or frequent nasal congestion are more likely to experience OSA. In some cases, medication can reduce snoring and open the airway for better nighttime breathing. Nasal strips also can reduce snoring. (Keep in mind that these treatments help breathing but do not treat OSA.)

Positive airway pressure therapy

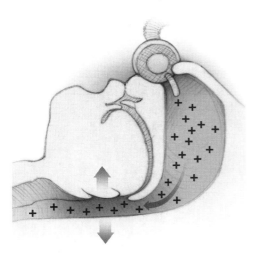

There are several types of positive airway pressure therapy: continuous (CPAP), bi-level (Bi-PAP), and automatic (APAP). Each delivers air from a machine through a mask, technically known as an interface, and into a patient's airway. This prevents nasal and throat passages from collapsing during sleep, therefore reducing apneic episodes. Air pressure is delivered in different manners depending on the type of machine; masks are available in many styles and sizes.

Personalizing PAP therapy to fit an individual's specific treatment needs is critical to the therapy's success. This is why a physician consultation and educational session prior to use are so important. A professional can assist patients in choosing the correct mask and brief them on what to expect with the treatment.

PAP therapy is a long-term solution for OSA, but some patients who do not allow time (up to two months) to adjust to the therapy abort the treatment before they can experience its benefits. Communication with a physician is especially important during the "training wheel" stages of PAP therapy. Tell your doctor if air pressure is too strong, if the mask chafes skin, or if the machine noise bothers a bed partner. There is a wide assortment of PAP equipment on the market. (And most of today's machines purr quietly and are not disruptive to sleep once patients and bed partners grow accustomed to the white noise.)

Proper "titration" is necessary for CPAP treatment. During this process, a sleep lab technologist will explain CPAP therapy and fit the patient with a comfortable mask or nasal cushions. A CPAP titration study is an overnight sleep study similar to the polysomnogram, in which sleep is recorded using the same electrodes and sensors but with the addition of PAP. The technologist will observe breathing and sleep quality, and increase or decrease settings during the night to determine which air pressure setting is best.

PAP treatment is effective in about 90 percent of patients who use machines most of the time, but education and titration to determine appropriate air pressure provide a critical success factor. After Dan was first diagnosed with OSA, he did not have a CPAP titration during the course of treatment. Therefore, his CPAP machine was probably not set at the appropriate pressure to abolish apnea episodes – and worse, the treatment was uncomfortable for him. This explains why he felt the treatment was "not really helping."

Common complaints among patients who use CPAP therapy include dry mouth, a leaking mask, sore or red eyes, nasal congestion, and skin irritation from the mask. Again, a consultation with a physician may prevent these aggravations or at least minimize them so the treatment is tolerable. CPAP can effectively control OSA as long as a patient commits to using it on a nightly basis.

Oral appliances

Patients with mild OSA might benefit from a device that advances the tongue or jaw forward to open the airway. Though this method is usually not sufficient for severe OSA, patients with minor cases who cannot tolerate CPAP therapy might respond to this alternative. However, not everyone is a good candidate for this approach. For example, patients without teeth (edentulous) and those with severe TMJ (temporomandibular junction) cannot use this approach. A sleep specialist and a dentist or prosthodontist with expertise in oral appliances for this purpose should jointly determine whether this treatment is best for you.

When it comes to dental appliances, once size doesn't fit all. That's why many specialists recommend adjustable devices. One example is the Klearway, which is an adjustable oral appliance that can be tailored to the anatomic needs of the individual. The OSA patient will adjust a crank on the device, say, every two weeks. This will expand the device and gradually advance the jaw forward.

Surgery

In recent years, the list of upper airway surgical procedures to treat snoring and sleep apnea has grown drastically. This includes minimally invasive approaches performed by an otolaryngologist (ear, nose, and throat specialist) in the office, such as somnoplasty, done to shrink excess tissue in the palate, uvula and tongue; laser-assisted uvuloplasty, which removes airway obstructions; tonsillectomy; nasal septoplasty, which straightens the nasal septum; and uvulopalatopharyngoplasty, which removes excess throat tissue to make the airway wider. Also available are more extensive procedures performed to reposition the jaw such as maxillary and mandibular advancement. Tracheostomy is rarely performed today, but it is exceedingly effective. This procedure involves creating a hole, or stoma, in the neck. A tube is inserted in the stoma to bypass the obstruction in the nose or throat. This is often reserved for life-threatening cases of OSA that do not respond to other therapies.

Before recommending any type of surgery, a sleep specialist and surgeon must determine whether the patient's goal is realistic. Some patients just snore. In this case, breaking and reforming the jaw is an extreme measure to stop the sound. On the other hand, somnoplasty cures snoring in nearly 100 percent of cases and is a less invasive solution. But if the patient weighs 300 pounds, a somnoplasty won't eliminate snoring or stop OSA. A physician will explain whether a procedure is necessary, conduct a risk assessment, and determine whether the surgery's results will meet the patient's desired outcome.

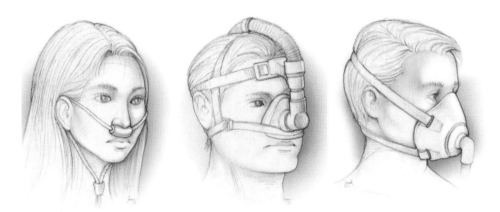

Dan's outcome

After the sleep study, a specialist evaluated Dan and gave him an educational session about OSA. Dan was fitted with a new mask and headgear (the straps and other essentials needed to keep the CPAP device securely in place during sleep). Dan was surprised at how many masks he could choose from. When he received his machine the first time, he recalls having it delivered with little education provided and no choice of mask type.

Dan learned how to maintain the equipment to keep it clean and minimize infections. His machine came equipped with a heated humidifier, and he was given a chinstrap to help keep his mouth closed at night. This way, the air forced through the mask would not escape through his mouth. He and Karen were counseled on the importance of using CPAP *all night, every night* to maximize its effect. Given that Dan's apnea is in the severe range, he is at risk for high blood pressure, heart attack, stroke, and diabetes should he fail to take this seriously.

After his follow-up visit a few weeks later, Dan started taking an occasional "night off" from the CPAP machine. Both he and Karen suffered the consequences: Karen couldn't sleep those nights; Dan had trouble staying awake the following days. He quickly learned that spending a few minutes before bed each night to secure the mask was a healthy choice for both of them.

Within the first year of treatment, Dan was able to resume an exercise program, using the time he had spent napping, and eventually lost some weight. He returns every year to the sleep clinic for reevaluation.

Chapter 6
Narcolepsy

Even where sleep is concerned, too much is a bad thing.

– Homer

Narcolepsy's *hallmark is excessive daytime sleepiness characterized by repeated episodes of "naps" or lapses into sleep.*

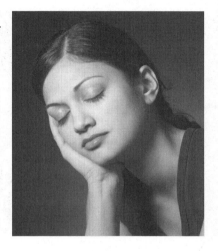

Falling asleep is never a concern for Felicia, who conks out moments after her head hits the pillow. Even if one of her typical bouts of acid reflux burns in her chest, she usually rolls over to her left side and easily slips back into a deep sleep until the alarm sounds at 5:30 a.m. Felicia likes to get to the office before the rest of her staff, and her workload as executive vice president of a marketing firm demands extra hours in the office.

Despite work stress, Felicia never has a problem falling asleep – she's like a rock each night. But strangely, she never feels rested. She figures this is because of her early wake-up call.

Lately, Felicia's days have been punctuated by "slips" when her mind and body check out. For example, sometimes while driving to work, she will hit a speed bump that jerks her out of a daze. She admits that her husband, Reynold, nudges her during car trips – even short ones – so she won't daydream or have a "head bob" at the wheel. He knows she works hard during the day, so he never questions her catnaps before dinner or her lazy Sundays. She may sleep on the couch for hours at a time if she doesn't have to run errands.

After prodding from Reynold, Felicia visited a doctor to discuss her fatigue and sluggishness. During a sleep interview, the doctor learned that she slept about nine hours each night, going to bed by 8:30 to 9 on work nights. The specialist asked Felicia about her sleep hygiene, daytime sleepiness, breathing, movements, and any habits she noticed during sleep. Felicia's weekdays are fairly routine. She fuels up with a cup of coffee at home and then stops at the coffee shop close to her office for a refill. She takes several coffee breaks throughout the morning.

By the time Felicia gets home at 5:30 p.m., she's exhausted after plugging away since 7 a.m. She and Reynold fix dinner and share a cup of tea, though Felicia usually dozes off in her chair and eventually retires to the bedroom.

Felicia's sleep assessment

Sleep snapshot

Felicia practices good sleep hygiene. She doesn't watch television, eat, or read in bed. She reports falling asleep immediately, waking up only to go to the bathroom or because of a sudden leg jerk or shortness of breath. She experiences reflux symptoms, but her heartburn has subsided since she quit smoking. She stopped having her nightly glass of red wine some years ago, as it usually made her feel even sleepier the next day.

Medical and family history

In addition to the reflux symptoms, Felicia has asthma. Her father has diabetes. Her grandmother had throat cancer. She says that sleep disorders do not run in her family, but she notes that her father snored and her mother often took naps during the day. Felicia had a great-aunt who slept excessively and told tales at family gatherings about her vivid dreams.

Excessive daytime sleepiness

Felicia admits she never feels refreshed in the morning, no matter how long and hard she sleeps. She sneaks in several catnaps a day and says she would sleep all day if she could. Drowsy driving is a concern. Felicia has never had a car accident or received a moving violation, but she can fall asleep during a stoplight and will roll down windows to stay refreshed, even on short drives.

Felicia took the Epworth Sleepiness Scale test, the questionnaire that measures daytime sleepiness. When the physician evaluated her test, her score was a 19, suggesting severe daytime sleepiness. Scores of 10 and higher are abnormal.

Insomnia

Felicia does not display signs of insomnia and says she had not experienced recent changes in life events. She says her bedroom is comfortable, and sleep onset is immediate. After learning about Felicia's sleep habits earlier, the doctor ruled out insomnia.

Narcolepsy

Felicia's high ESS score and complaints of daytime sleepiness struck a chord with the physician. When asked whether she ever felt weak in her legs, arms, or jaw when she felt strong emotions, Felicia told a story that led to her diagnosis.

"Have you ever lost control over your body when you were laughing at a joke or were angry?" the physician asked Felicia.

"Like when my dog pees on the carpet?"

"What happens then?"

"I get so mad that I can't talk or move." Felicia told the doctor that she has even reached out to scold the dog, lost muscle control in her legs, and dropped to her knees.

Perfect cataplexy, the doctor thought to herself. Cataplexy is an abrupt decrease in or loss of muscle tone, and it is frequently elicited by laughter, anger, or surprise. It can occur in more than two-thirds of patients with narcolepsy. Typically during a cataplectic episode, the jaw sags, head falls forward, arms drop to the side, and the knees unlock or buckle. Severity ranges from complete paralysis to limited muscle loss to a quick sensation of weakness.

Physicians sometimes overlook short cataplectic attacks, like those described by Felicia, because they do not occur during sleep studies and they do not resemble full-blown attacks.

The diagnosis

From time to time, Felicia also displays sleep paralysis. Common in patients with narcolepsy, this behavior occurs when the brain is awake, but the body remains in the motionless state characteristic of REM. Their mind says, "Move!" But their body resists. This conflict is scary and confusing for patients.

Considering Felicia's excessive daytime sleepiness, cataplectic behavior, reports of occasional sleep paralysis, and excessive use of caffeine, the doctor determined that she might have a disorder known as narcolepsy with cataplexy. She ordered Felicia not to drive until after an overnight sleep study and multiple sleep latency test.

During the overnight study, people with narcolepsy also may present with symptoms of sleep apnea or other disorders. However, more often, narcoleptics show disruptions in normal sleep patterns with frequent awakenings not explained by apnea. During an MSLT, the patient takes five nap trials at two-hour intervals, beginning ninety minutes to three hours after the morning awakening. Narcoleptics generally fall asleep at every opportunity, often in less than five minutes, while normal people stay awake the entire time or fall asleep no sooner than ten minutes after each trial starts. In addition, most people with narcolepsy fall quickly into REM sleep, known as sleep-onset REM periods. Felicia's MSLT and polysomnogram (PSG) demonstrated all these features, with a mean sleep latency (the average time to fall asleep across five nap trials) of 4.6 minutes. Sleep-onset REM periods occurred during two of the five trials.

After reviewing results from the PSG and MSLT, the doctor diagnosed Felicia with narcolepsy and prescribed a stimulant.

All about narcolepsy

The profile – is this you?

A common complaint of narcoleptics is that a twenty-minute nap is refreshing, but a couple of hours later, they are sleepy again. Bosses often view narcoleptics as lazy and unmotivated, especially if they know of frequent naps and observe extreme sleepiness on the job. Relationships with spouses and family members also can suffer, as narcoleptics seem lethargic or uninterested when really they are exhausted beyond their control.

Narcoleptics often learn to cope with the disease. In fact, most have learned how to work, play, and live with sleepiness because they grew up tired. Narcolepsy can range in severity, with some patients regarding sleepiness as an inconvenient nuisance that has them dozing during conversations or falling asleep in situations that do not require active participation. On the other hand, narcolepsy for some is a life-threatening illness, especially in cases where patients fall asleep while operating automobiles or heavy machinery. These patients display sudden, uncontrollable sleep attacks during active situations in which normal sleep never occurs – while eating, walking, driving, or attending interactive meetings.

Symptoms

Excessive daytime sleepiness is the main symptom of narcolepsy, and it generally surfaces in the early teen years and 20s. Narcolepsy is less likely in older adults but can begin at any age. Many of the features of narcolepsy are due to the abnormal tendency of patients to slip almost instantly from wakefulness into REM sleep.

Symptoms of narcolepsy include:

- Excessive daytime sleepiness, usually the first symptom

- Recurrent daytime naps or lapses into sleep that occur almost daily for at least three months

- Disturbed sleep

- Automatic behavior; continuation of apparently normal behavior like taking a test or driving, without memory or awareness.

- Pathological manifestations of REM sleep (such as cataplexy, sleep paralysis, and hypnagogic hallucinations)

Cataplexy: In this state, narcoleptics experience a sudden loss of muscle tone provoked by laughter, joking, surprise, or anger; consciousness remains clear, memory is not impaired, and respiration is intact, although the patient cannot speak or respond. Cataplexy usually lasts a few seconds to several minutes, and patients recover gradually over a few minutes. A patient can suffer from daytime sleepiness and present symptoms of narcolepsy but not experience cataplexy for up to thirty years. Cataplexy rarely precedes sleepiness. The frequency of attacks varies from a few in a lifetime to many per day. Some patients avoid emotional situations for fear of a cataplectic attack.

Sleep paralysis: This is a transient inability to move or speak during the transition between sleep and wakefulness. Sleep paralysis is often paired with a sensation of inability to breathe, which frightens patients. Most narcoleptics experience sleep paralysis; episodes usually resolve in a couple of minutes. They occur in 40 to 80 percent of narcoleptics.

Hypnagogic hallucinations: These are vivid perceptual experiences that occur at sleep onset (or in the transition from sleep to wakefulness, in which case they are called hypnopompic hallucinations), generally with awareness of the presence of a person or thing. Patients might describe hallucinations such as running from danger, flying through the air, or feeling as if someone or something is touching them. Often, hypnogogic hallucinations include abnormal perceptions of sight, sound, movements, and touch. They are about as common as sleep paralysis in narcoleptics.

A PSG and MSLT of a narcolepsy patient will reveal one or more of the following symptoms:

- Sleep latency of less than ten minutes (time it takes to fall asleep).

- REM sleep latency of less than twenty minutes (sleep-onset REM period) on the polysomnogram.

- Increased amount of stage 1 sleep and frequent arousals and awakenings.

- A mean sleep latency on the MSLT of less than eight minutes, usually less than five minutes, and two or more sleep-onset REM periods. However, up to 25 percent of narcoleptics may lack these findings.

Other factors that can confirm a narcolepsy diagnosis

Low hypocretin levels

Cells in the hypothalamus, deep in the brain, regulate wakefulness. These cells secrete a peptide called hypocretin. When researchers performed spinal taps to extract cerebrospinal fluid (CSF) of narcolepsy patients (as might be done to evaluate for meningitis), they discovered a deficiency in hypocretin. In the last couple of years, such studies have sparked ideas that narcolepsy is a degenerative process that destroys hypocretin, which keeps a person awake. This hypothesis would explain why narcoleptics fall asleep; they lack a substance in their brains that tells the body to stay awake. Low (CSF) hypocretin levels are seen in 90 percent of patients with narcolepsy and cataplexy, but almost never in healthy people or patients with daytime sleepiness due to other disorders.

Family history

The risk of developing narcolepsy is 1 to 2 percent in first-degree relatives of narcoleptics. Narcoleptics also have a higher risk of obesity and Type 2 diabetes mellitus, which may relate to dysfunction in the hypocretin-secreting cells of the hypothalamus.

Felicia's aunt displayed characteristics of narcolepsy, though she was never formally diagnosed with the disorder. Her father's history of diabetes puts Felicia at risk for this disease as well.

Excessive daytime sleepiness and hypersomnia

Felicia's symptoms clearly signified that she has narcolepsy with cataplexy. (Some narcoleptic patients do not have cataplexy, which may cause more difficulty in diagnosing the disorder.) Hypersomnia is the opposite of insomnia – hypersomniacs sleep a lot and still feel sleepy. Because our society does not always recognize serious sleepiness as a medical issue, many people who suffer from hypersomnia write it off as just being "really tired." While sleeping more is effective in reducing daytime sleepiness, some patients have an underlying disorder not helped by earlier bedtimes and more time allocated to sleep.

Hypersomniacs may display symptoms similar to those of narcoleptics during an MSLT – low sleep latency and an occasional sleep-onset REM period. This is why keeping a sleep log prior to sleep lab testing is extremely critical for a proper diagnosis. Sleep logs will help physicians rule out unusual sleep-wake cycles causing hypersomnia. This log also will show how much sleep is "normal" for the individual so physicians can compare sleeping habits to overnight PSG and MSLT results.

Patients may be asked to perform a urine drug screen the morning of the MSLT to rule out drug use as a cause of hypersomnia. Medications that suppress REM sleep, such as stimulants and antidepressants, should be discontinued before the study; a period of two weeks off such medications is recommended.

Excessive daytime sleepiness or narcolepsy?

Following are some questions your physician might ask you to determine the cause and severity of excessive daytime sleepiness.

1. Do you feel sleepy no matter how much sleep you get?

2. Do you fall asleep in inappropriate situations or find yourself fighting to stay awake while driving or in meetings, even after a full night's sleep?

3. Do you experience spells of muscle weakness when you are happy, sad, or angry?

4. Do you dream during short naps?

5. Do your family or friends describe situations in which your sleepiness was unusual or memorable? (Many narcoleptics were the joke of their family on trips and family events.)

6. Do you use caffeine excessively to stay awake (including No-Doz, Mountain Dew, etc.)?

7. Do you find yourself in places without knowing how you got there or have you lost time in the middle of a task?

8. Do you snore or wake up gasping for air?

9. Do you have uncomfortable sensations in your legs at night that are relieved by stretching or walking?

10. Do you sleep much longer on weekends than during the week?

If you answered yes to the first seven questions, you may have narcolepsy.

If you snore regularly, explore the possibility of sleep apnea. You could be diagnosed with both narcolepsy and sleep apnea if symptoms of both are evident through your polysomnogram and sleep questionnaires.

Restless legs syndrome is a common disorder in which unusual leg sensations interfere with one's ability to fall asleep or stay asleep. (We will address this further in Chapter 7.)

Finally, if you sleep in much later on weekends than on weekdays, your body is simply refueling its stores from insufficient sleep during the week. Insufficient sleep syndrome, rampant in modern society, is the most common cause of daytime sleepiness.

Felicia's outcome

Felicia was diagnosed with narcolepsy with cataplexy and instructed on the importance of maintaining strict bedtime and wake times, including on weekends. The physician warned her to avoid all drugs (including alcohol) that depress the central nervous system and contribute to daytime sleepiness. She was instructed to take at least two scheduled naps daily to ward off unscheduled sleep episodes. For many narcoleptics, five-minute catnaps are extraordinarily effective.

Following these simple measures, Felicia was prescribed the stimulant medication Provigil (modafinil, 200 mg) upon awakening to improve alertness. This initial dose had only a modest effect and was gradually increased to 600 mg per day. Excessive daytime sleepiness improved, but cataplexy continued.

How to get a good night's sleep

Narcolepsy: Provigil is a stimulant used to treat excessive sleepiness associated with narcolepsy, obstructive sleep apnea, and shift work sleep disorder (read more about this in Chapter 11.) It increases a patient's ability to maintain wakefulness, although it may not stop all sleepiness. It may improve wakefulness in patients with daytime sleepiness due to other disorders.

As with any stimulant, users should know that side effects are similar to those of being overcaffeinated: agitation, nervousness, and palpitations. Start with a low dose and very slowly work up to a larger dose, as tolerance develops over time with some agents.

Here is a list of commonly prescribed stimulants* that can be used to treat excessive daytime sleepiness:

- Ritalin
- Adderall
- Concerta
- Dexedrine
- Focalin
- Metadate

These are brand names

The use of wakefulness-promoting agents has been associated with high blood pressure and heart arrhythmias. People taking these medications should be closely monitored.

Cataplexy: In the 1970s and 1980s, cataplexy was treated primarily with tricyclic antidepressants (TCAs); they were not effective in all cases and produced a lot of side effects. Selective serotonin reuptake inhibitors (SSRIs) came on the scene and were as effective with fewer side effects than TCAs. The U.S. Food and Drug Administration approved the first drug – Xyrem – for cataplexy in 2002. Xyrem's history is recreational – it was abused as a date-rape drug, which explains why the substance is tightly controlled and available in the U.S. only through a single central pharmacy. However, Xyrem is purported to reduce severe cataplexy by 85 percent while improving excessive daytime sleepiness. Xyrem also improves the fragmented sleep of narcoleptics.

Chapter 7
Restless Legs Syndrome

Life is something that happens when you can't get to sleep.

– Fran Lebowitz

Restless legs syndrome *is characterized by a strong, often irresistible urge to move the legs. This is often accompanied by sensations such as tingling, numbness, or pain. Symptoms usually begin in the evening and are relieved by moving, stretching, or rubbing the legs.*

Maria settles into her favorite reclining chair to unwind each night with every intention of zoning out into a relaxed state. She finishes a few more chapters in her book and channel-surfs until she lands on a sitcom that requires as much brainpower as she has left after a long day. Eventually, Maria's tension melts and her body begins to relax.

But her legs are hardly at ease.

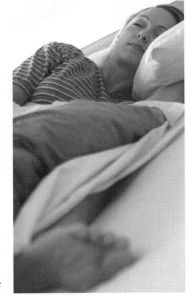

The last couple of years, Maria has experienced uncomfortable sensations in her lower limbs. Her legs ache and tingle until she massages them, flexes her calves, or finally gets up and walks around her living room. Like clockwork, when her brain turns off for the day, her legs turn on – and lately, she's noticed that the cramping surfaces for a minute or two during the day as well.

Once Maria retires to bed, the bothersome feeling prevents her from falling asleep and wakes her up several times during the night. The sensations stop only when she shimmies her lower half, wiggles her toes, or gets out of bed and paces around the room. Her husband jokingly calls her "Twinkle Toes" because he feels her restless legs and hears her feet pitter-patter throughout the night.

Maria's sleep assessment

Sleep snapshot

Once a sound sleeper, Maria developed insomnia two years ago with the onset of menopause. In the last six months, her condition has gotten worse. Her sleep is variable; she goes to bed anytime from 8:30 to 11 p.m. and usually spends one hour tossing and turning before she falls asleep. She wakes up at least five times during the night. She assumes she must have to go to the bathroom, but she usually finds that her legs are uncomfortable and she must stretch or move them. Sometimes, she awakens with hot flashes, although these have significantly lessened lately. Frustrated, Maria finally starts her day between 5 and 9 a.m. Her average five to six hours of sleep is far less than the eight to nine hours she got just five years ago. Because her nights are filled with frequent interruptions, she feels as if she never actually sleeps.

Excessive daytime sleepiness

Maria usually drags out of bed every weekday morning to get ready for work. A nap is a luxury she usually can't afford, but sometimes she'll sneak in a short one – even a quick ten to twenty minutes during lunch break.

Insomnia

Maria has been taking prescription sleeping pills to calm her insomnia symptoms, and due to a significant amount of stress, she says her sleeplessness is worse and she relies more on the medication. She takes it when she feels "really bad," which is at least once a week.

Medical and family history

Maria does not report a family history of narcolepsy, sleep apnea, or other sleep disorders. However, she says her mother complained of feelings in her legs that kept her up at night.

The diagnosis

Maria's physician ordered a polysomnogram so he could better understand the cause of her nighttime awakenings. He diagnosed her with restless legs syndrome (RLS). Maria's family history of RLS increased the likelihood by up to ten times that she might also have the disorder. Also, the time in which Maria's legs bother her – early evening and during the night – is consistent with symptoms of RLS.

All about restless legs syndrome

Because RLS symptoms are often difficult to describe and may occur only once or twice per month at first, many people forget to bring up the subject to a doctor or they figure that tingling legs are due to a pinched nerve from a particular body position or leg cramps. Others attribute the sensation to arthritis pain, vascular problems, or nervous system problems. (Diabetics and people on dialysis for kidney failure are particularly prone to RLS.) As for children who complain of achy legs, their parents might explain away the sensations as just growing pains. On top of this, patients might not recognize that tingling legs can trigger insomnia. When you aren't comfortable, you don't sleep.

Leg cramps or "charley horses" (those sharp calf pains usually attributed to sore muscles or a mineral deficiency) are different from restless legs syndrome. RLS patients have a strong urge to move legs at night – an urge they cannot resist. The feeling generally subsides in the morning, though patients with severe conditions report that sensations occasionally flare up during the day as well. The urge is often accompanied by a feeling of burning, itching, prickling, tingling, or aching, and the discomfort can range from mild to severe. Temporary relief comes only with moving the legs.

Leg muscles also might tighten or flex while a patient is still. Repetitive muscle movements of the lower extremities, known as periodic limb movements (PLMs), can occur during the night, arousing the patient and reducing quality of sleep. These movements also can occur while the patient is awake in bed. PLMs take center stage in another closely related disorder, known as periodic limb movement disorder (PLMD), which is characterized by periodic, repetitive limb movements during sleep that lead to insomnia or daytime sleepiness.

PLMD and RLS are two different sleep disorders. However, symptoms sometimes overlap, and about 85 percent of patients with RLS report involuntary leg jerking or twitching either during sleep or awake while sitting or lying in bed. Patients with only PLMD do not experience the type of sensations or level of discomfort associated with RLS.

Who gets RLS?

RLS has been described as the most common disorder no one has heard of. Five to 10 percent of Caucasians in the world are affected. The disorder is rare among Asian populations. RLS is more common in women than in men, and it affects individuals of all ages. Those who develop RLS before age 45 are considered "early-onset" cases and often have relatives affected with the disorder. These patients experience symptoms slowly over time. Once a person is 45 to

65 years old, RLS can set in suddenly and progress quickly. A patient might feel leg sensations every night from the day RLS starts.

More than 50 percent of patients with the disorder are diagnosed with primary or idiopathic RLS, meaning their restless legs are not associated with other medical problems. Many patients also report family histories of RLS or report a parent who experienced unusual sensations and discomfort in the lower extremities. The chance of developing RLS increases ten-fold when an immediate relative has the disorder.

RLS and its relationship with other medical disorders

A laundry list of medical problems as well as medications can provoke RLS. There are links between the disorder and iron deficiency, Parkinson's disease, renal disease, diabetes, and peripheral neuropathy (a nervous system disease). Pregnant women often note symptoms of RLS typically after twenty weeks of gestation, and dialysis patients are especially susceptible to developing RLS. Patients who take antidepressants, sedating antihistamines, or virtually any centrally active dopamine-receptor antagonist (such as anti-nausea medication) are candidates for secondary RLS.

In many of these cases, RLS is a temporary disorder that is resolved when other conditions are treated. But when RLS regularly disturbs sleep, specific treatment methods are necessary.

How do you know you have RLS?

The hallmark of RLS is an intense, irresistible urge to move the legs, often accompanied by other sensations in the legs that may be difficult for a person to describe. Certain criteria are necessary to make an RLS diagnosis. Patients must answer yes to the following questions:

1. Do you have the urge to move the extremities, usually accompanied by uncomfortable or unpleasant sensations in the legs?

2. Do you have the urge to move or have uncomfortable sensations that begin or worsen during periods of rest or inactivity?

3. Do you have the urge to move or have uncomfortable sensations that are partially or totally relieved by movement, such as walking or stretching?

4. Do you have the urge to move or have uncomfortable sensations that are worse or occur solely in the evening or at night?

Some exceptions to these criteria are as follows:

- The patient previously met criteria and has undergone a spontaneous remission or is participating in a drug study with subsequent significant alteration of symptoms.

- The patient at one time got relief of symptoms by activity, but discomfort now is so severe that relief is impossible.

- The patient at one time was worse later in the day or at night, but symptoms now are so severe that they are equal day and night.

If a patient presents with RLS based on these criteria, a physician may use a standardized questionnaire to grade the severity, known as the International RLS Rating Scale. Patients circle the rating that describes how they felt **in the past week**. Physicians add up the numbers to determine severity. (*See scale at end of test.*)

1. Overall, how would you rate the <u>RLS discomfort in your legs or arms</u>?
   (4) Very severe
   (3) Severe
   (2) Moderate
   (1) Mild
   (0) None

2. Overall, how would you rate the <u>need to move</u> around because of your RLS symptoms?
   (4) Very severe
   (3) Severe
   (2) Moderate
   (1) Mild
   (0) None

3. Overall, how much <u>relief of</u> your RLS arm or leg discomfort do you get from moving around?
   (4) No relief
   (3) Mild relief
   (2) Moderate relief
   (1) Either complete or almost complete relief
   (0) No RLS symptoms to be relieved

4. How severe was your <u>sleep disturbance</u> due to your RLS symptoms?
   (4) Very severe
   (3) Severe
   (2) Moderate
   (1) Mild
   (0) None

5. How severe was your <u>tiredness</u> or <u>sleepiness</u> during the day due to your RLS symptoms?
   (4) Very severe
   (3) Severe
   (2) Moderate
   (1) Mild
   (0) None

6. How severe was <u>your RLS as a whole</u>?
   (4) Very severe
   (3) Severe
   (2) Moderate
   (1) Mild
   (0) None

7. How <u>often</u> did you get RLS symptoms?
   (4) Very often (6 to 7 days a week)
   (3) Often (4 to 5 days a week)
   (2) Sometimes (2 to 3 days a week)
   (1) Occasionally (1 day a week)
   (0) Never

8. When you had RLS symptoms, how severe were they on average?
   (4) Very severe (8 hours or more per 24-hour day)
   (3) Severe (3 to 8 hours per 24-hour day)
   (2) Moderate (1 to 3 hours per 24-hour day)
   (1) Mild (less than 1 hour per 24-hour day)
   (0) None

9. <u>Overall</u>, how severe was the impact of your RLS symptoms on your ability to carry out your <u>daily affairs</u> – for example, carrying out a satisfactory family, home, social, school, or work life?
   (4) Very severe
   (3) Severe
   (2) Moderate
   (1) Mild
   (0) None

10. How severe was your <u>mood disturbance</u> from your RLS symptoms – for example, angry, depressed, sad, anxious or irritable?
   (4) Very severe
   (3) Severe
   (2) Moderate
   (1) Mild
   (0) None

Severity Scale:

Very Severe	=	31-40 points
Severe	=	21-30 points
Moderate	=	11-20 points
Mild	=	1-10 points
None	=	0 points

How to get a good night's sleep

A regular exercise program can reduce symptoms of RLS in patients with mild cases. Movement during the day has been shown to ease leg sensations in the evening. While sitting, patients with less advanced RLS can reduce symptoms by staying mentally active.

Additionally, these general measures can lessen RLS symptoms:

- Reduce caffeine intake
- Limit use of alcohol
- Stop smoking
- Eliminate drugs known to cause RLS

When RLS occurs, the following activities can help alleviate leg sensations:

- Walking
- Riding an exercise bike
- Massaging or rubbing lower leg area
- Soaking in a hot tub

Since iron deficiency is a reversible cause of RLS, many sleep specialists recommend over-the-counter iron tablets (ferrous sulfate). A simple blood test can measure iron stores in the body and help physicians determine who might benefit from iron therapy.

Medications

Physicians can treat RLS with dopaminergic drugs that replace dopamine, a neurotransmitter in the brain. Also used to treat conditions such as Parkinson's disease, these drugs control the urge to move and sensory symptoms and reduce involuntary leg jerking in sleep. Currently, ropinirole (Requip) is the only FDA-approved drug for RLS although several drugs with dopaminergic action, including levodopa, are effective.

There are four classes of drugs prescribed to treat RLS:

Dopaminergic drugs: These are the primary therapies used to treat moderate to severe RLS in patients who are unresponsive to non-drug interventions. In addition to ropinirole, pramiprexole, pergolide, and levodopa are effective.

Anti-seizure medications: These control sensations by slowing or blocking pain signals from nerves. Examples include gabapentin and carbamazepine. Gabapentin is particularly effective in patients with painful RLS related to peripheral nervous system disorders.

Benzodiazepines: Sometimes prescribed for mild RLS, these drugs are criticized by some physicians for their addictive potential and side effects like daytime drowsiness. Clonazepam and temazepam fall into this category.

Opioids: These "pain killer" drugs are used to alleviate aching and uncomfortable sensations in legs; they are usually reserved for more severe cases that are not controlled with other agents and in painful RLS due to their potential for addiction. Many opioids are available. These are controlled substances that usually require a special type of prescription. Examples include codeine, oxycodone, and morphine, reserved for the most severe cases.

Maria's outcome

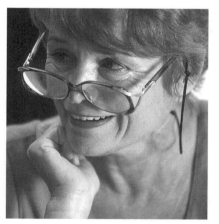

The diagnosis of RLS is made using the sleep history and overnight sleep testing is not necessarily required. Maria was referred to the sleep lab to evaluate repeated awakenings she experienced nearly every night. Maria's overnight sleep study demonstrated a delayed sleep onset during which she squirmed and exercised her legs in bed, trying to relieve the sensation. Periods of leg stretching were punctuated by involuntary leg jerks. Once asleep, her legs continued to jerk repeatedly in light sleep and during the transition from wakefulness to sleep. Movements lessened in deep NREM sleep and were absent in REM sleep.

The physician ordered a serum ferritin level to rule out iron deficiency, which was normal. He then recommended a trial of ropinirole, beginning with one pill at 8 p.m., since her leg movements would usually start by 10 p.m. (One major problem that often leads to incomplete response to treatment is that medications are often taken too late in the evening. Patients with symptoms in the early evening should take their first dose of medication at dinnertime.)

Maria's doctor increased the dose gradually, which virtually abolished all symptoms and improved the quality of her sleep. He warned her of the possibility of developing augmentation, a phenomenon in which symptoms of RLS begin earlier in the day due to the treatment. This is observed only with dopaminergic medications, most notably with levodopa. He also warned her about unusual side effects, including sudden sleep attacks and melanoma, a rare complication of dopaminergic therapy observed in patients with Parkinson's disease.

Chapter 8
Psychophysiological Insomnia

> *Insomnia is a gross feeder. It will nourish itself on any kind of thinking, including thinking about not thinking.*
>
> *— Clifton Fadiman*

Psychophysiological insomnia *occurs when a patient responds to stress or other environmental conditions with tension. The patient learns sleep-preventing associations, which result in difficulty falling and staying asleep.*

Ann recalls her worst string of sleepless nights – forty in a row. She dreads "lights out," knowing that she probably won't nod off until at least 2 a.m. So she worries and gives herself a pep talk every night before bed. *Tonight, you can sleep,* she tells herself. *But what if I can't sleep? How long will I stay awake tonight? How can I lose sleep another night? It's already getting late…*

Once in bed, Ann lies awake, subtracting each passing hour from the sleep total she will achieve before her 6 o'clock wake-up call for work. It's a numbers game for Ann, and the more minutes she counts, the more sleep she loses. While she's awake, she can't stop thinking about her sick in-laws, her work responsibilities, and her changing body, which won't let her feel "normal." *How will I hold it all together?* she frets.

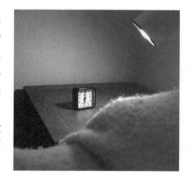

Before this particular bout of insomnia, Ann's doctor had changed her sleeping-pill prescription. This new medication wasn't working, and Ann wrote off her insomnia to not being able to adjust to the different prescription. Ann had been anxious about the switch. But then, she was uneasy about a lot of things in her life these days.

Ann, 46, has complained of insomnia for the last six years. Symptoms of peri-menopause and related physical changes disrupt her sleep; hot flashes or night sweats wake her from time to time. But lately, the wakefulness has lasted two to three hours on "really bad" nights. During a sleep assessment, Ann mentioned that a few years ago she was treated for depression. When the physician pressed her for details, Ann said she had worked through that period of her life.

Ann has taken some steps to improve her sleep environment. She removed the television from her bedroom – a distraction that can trigger insomnia. Also, she established a nighttime ritual. The problem: Her disruptive sleep is also a regular pattern, and Ann estimates that she sleeps only four hours each night.

Insomnia and sleep insecurity

Besides anxiety, depression, or underlying psychological disorders already present in many patients diagnosed with various types of insomnia, patients like Ann develop a fear of not falling asleep. They worry each night. *What if I can't fall asleep? How will I function at my meeting tomorrow on two hours of rest? Will tonight be as bad as last night?* Then they might turn on the television while in bed or feverishly check the glaring, digitized numbers on their clocks. Sleep insecurity grows with every toss and turn, with every night of lost sleep.

Like most patients who exhibit symptoms of insomnia, Ann subscribes to a similar nightly pattern. Her insomnia was first triggered by stress and physical change: pre-menopause, difficulties in her marriage, ill family members. While some people react to tension by getting headaches, stomachaches, or other physical maladies, other people like Ann respond by not sleeping.

Once sleep loss occurs every night, a patient's ability to function during the day suffers. People feed their own disorder by developing habits that disrupt sleep. Essentially, the insecurity that diagnosed insomniacs feel when they try to sleep worsens the disorder and increases their sleep deficit. They are not relaxed in the evening, they watch television or read in bed to fall asleep, and they are distracted and awake during the night. Because they are tired during the day, they turn to caffeine and other stimulants, which can trigger wakefulness hours after the substances are consumed. It becomes a vicious cycle.

By considering how day and night behaviors and activities affect sleep and a patient's perception of sleep, physicians can better understand causes and treat the disorder. Physical and psychiatric factors, lifestyle, and environment all factor into a patient's inability to sleep.

Ann's sleep assessment

Sleep snapshot

Ann spends eight hours in bed each night, but she thinks only four are spent sleeping; she estimates that she needs eight hours to function properly. She goes to bed at 10 p.m. and wakes up at 6 each morning. She maintains a relatively consistent sleep schedule on weekends, indulging in several extra hours in bed on Saturdays and Sundays, but during this time she rarely does more than rest. Ann avoids eating, watching television, or reading in bed. She knows that poor

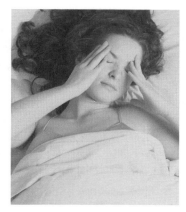

"sleep hygiene" will only worsen her ability to sleep at night. She always wakes up several times per night, sometimes every hour on the hour. Just before and during her menstrual period, she usually spends at least one night entirely sleepless, or so it seems.

Ann takes a prescription sleeping pill as needed at bedtime. In fact, she has seen several physicians for her sleep problem and has taken just about every prescription sleeping pill on the market. Most didn't work for more than a couple of days, but Ann is afraid to go without her nightly pill. It has become a security blanket. She also takes a number of vitamins, including calcium, vitamins C, B, and E, and a soy supplement.

Excessive daytime sleepiness

Ann never feels refreshed. She is always tired and fatigued, and she couldn't nap during the day if her life depended on it. She is growing more concerned that her sleep loss will become apparent to her boss or that she'll fall asleep driving. She also worries that her sleepless nights are jeopardizing her health. She wonders how long a human being can survive without sleep.

Restless legs syndrome

Once a month, Ann develops an ache in her calf that increases when she puts weight on her legs. This can happen day or night, but she usually controls the pain by applying a heating pad to the area or doing squats to stretch her lower leg muscles. Nevertheless, the sensation is uncomfortable and can inhibit sleep. Ann has never been treated for an iron deficiency, which is associated with uncomfortable legs and restless legs syndrome.

Narcolepsy

Ann does not nap during the day, and though she often is worn out from restless nights, she is alert and scored a 4 on the Epworth Sleepiness Scale. (Remember, Felicia's score was 19; she had narcolepsy. Scores of 10 and higher indicate daytime sleepiness.)

Insomnia

When the physician asked Ann about recent changes or life events, he learned about Ann's family trauma and related stresses that keep her awake at night. Ann denies being depressed, though she said hormonal changes have made her anxious lately. The emotional activity in Ann's life spurred the doctor to explore potential psychophysiological insomnia, which develops because of two factors: somatized tension (muscle movement) and perpetuating behaviors that are sleep disruptive (ruminating, worrying, etc.). Her Fatigue Severity Score is 56 out of a maximum of 63, indicating a pronounced degree of fatigue and lack of energy.

Bruxism, or grinding teeth

Ann's husband noticed that she grinds her teeth some nights. Ann has a mouth guard, but she often does not wear it. If her jaw hurts in the morning, she will rub the area, take some ibuprofen, or use a heating pad. Her teeth grinding worsens during stressful times. This type of nervous activity is not unusual for insomniacs.

Medical and family history

Ann is healthy, though she exhibited some atypical chest pain a couple of years ago. This pain was a normal reaction to stress. She says her family does not have a history of narcolepsy, restless legs syndrome, or insomnia. She told the physician that her father died when she was 13 years old.

The diagnosis

Ann is shouldering a great deal of stress in her life, her body is going through mid-life change, and her emotions are responding to these internal and external factors through anxiety. Pulled in several directions, Ann is like many women who try to "hold it all together." Women are more likely to have insomnia than men, and women in Ann's age group are even more susceptible to the sleep disorder, as their hormones affect their ability to get a good night's sleep.

When the physician learned about Ann's history of depression, he questioned whether this was still an issue. Ann said that problems in her marriage five years ago prompted her to see a psychologist to discuss ways to cope with the tension. She took a prescription for a short time. However, because Ann has a history of emotional instability, the physician linked this past with her response to family challenges today. Ann isn't losing sleep because of idiopathic insomnia, which is a lifelong insomnia not caused by stress or emotional disturbances. She has experienced difficulty falling asleep only in recent years, so the physician knew that her disorder was not developed during childhood as a result of an inadequately developed sleep system or neurological disorder.

Rather, Ann's insomnia flared because of psychological and physical reasons. The physician's clinical impression for Ann was that she suffered from psychophysiological insomnia. The root of Ann's sleeping problems is not intrinsic, but rather a reaction to outside influences. Ann's restless sleep is learned, the physician told her. It can be treated by cognitive behavioral therapy and improved sleep hygiene.

Why Can't I Sleep?

There are universal triggers that keep people awake at night.

Medical conditions, even temporary ones such as a sprained ankle, sports injury, or minor surgery, can prevent sound sleep; so can chronic problems, such as heartburn, asthma, heart disease, and arthritis.

Life changes (a baby, a new spouse, a new job) also figure into the sleep equation. Many of these changes are exciting or present new challenges. Until you settle comfortably into new relationships and roles, sleep can suffer.

Emotions can inhibit sleep. When we feel frustration or hurt, anticipation, or even happiness, we tend to stay awake long past bedtime. Divorce, major illness, lawsuits, and bad investments churn negative emotions and promote anxiety – not states of mind that lead to relaxation and restful nights.

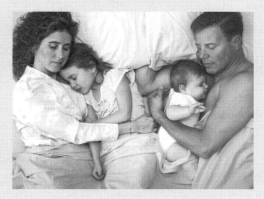

All about insomnia

How do you know if you have insomnia?

- Does it take you an excessively long period to fall asleep?

- Do you wake frequently? If so, do you have a difficult time falling back asleep?

- Do you try hard to fall asleep at night, but notice you easily can fall asleep during monotonous activities, such as watching television or reading?

- Do you watch television, read, or eat in bed?

- Are you a worrywart? Does your mind race at night thinking about your problems, the next day's schedule, or worries about sleep loss?

- Do you experience increased muscle tension or agitation (i.e., somatized tension) or inability to relax at night?

- Have you experienced a recent life change or emotional stress?

- Do you feel anxious or depressed?

- Do you complain of not sleeping or do you grow tired, irritable, or feel a deterioration of mood or motivation during the day?

When should I seek help?

If you answer yes to any number of these questions, consider visiting a physician to discuss sleep patterns and solutions. The physician will ask you to maintain a sleep log in which you track bedtimes, hours asleep, and how you feel during the day. This is important to learn how your sleep compares with "normal" sleep.

Also, if your sleep has been disrupted for more than a month and interferes with the way you function during the day, you should investigate these sleep patterns by talking to your physician or asking for a referral to see a sleep disorders specialist.

What causes insomnia?

Most people experience brief periods in their lives when they can't sleep – this is normal. But when behavior persists for a month or longer, and lack of sleep interferes with a person's ability to function during the day, the problem is more serious and warrants changes in lifestyle or cognitive behavioral therapy. First, physicians must understand the cause of insomnia, and several reasons – intrinsic and extrinsic – cause people to lose sleep.

Diet

Caffeinated substances, such as coffee, tea, soda, and chocolate, over-the-counter wakefulness-promoting agents, and some prescription drugs, stimulate the nervous system and may cause difficulty falling asleep or awakenings at night. This is not to say you should take your morning coffee off the breakfast menu or forget your late-afternoon chocolate. Moderate use during the day will not affect sleep onset in the evening for most people if they curb use several hours before bedtime. If you suffer from insomnia, limit caffeinated beverages and avoid drinking caffeine after noon. Excessive caffeine use can lead to withdrawal symptoms, which can affect one's ability to sleep.

Nicotine is another sleep-inhibiting stimulant. Smokers who break their habit might experience withdrawal symptoms at first, but once their body adjusts, they will find that they wake up less and sleep more soundly at night. If you can't quit the habit entirely, avoid smoking in the evening and absolutely during the night.

And, despite the theory that a "nightcap" is just the elixir for a good night's sleep, alcoholic beverages actually interfere with the body's ability to maintain deep sleep, which refreshes the body. Alcohol might induce sleep at first, but regular users are likely to wake up frequently and often report feeling drowsy and sleep-deprived in the morning.

Full meals before bedtime can trigger heartburn and stomachache – two reasons to eat heavy meals no later than four hours before going to sleep. A light snack, on the other hand, can promote sleep. Milk or cheese and crackers are good bedtime snacks.

Environment: Your bedroom

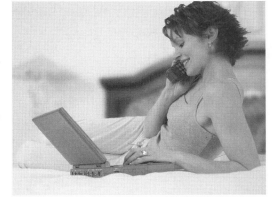

Some insomniacs set themselves up for a sleepless night before they even retire to their bedrooms. Rather than a calming oasis that invites sleep and relaxation, their bedrooms are activity centers equipped with televisions, computers, stereos, books, magazines, and other distractions. Their windows don't close out noise from a crowded street, their homes are positioned under a flight path, a train passes every day at 3 a.m., or they can hear their apartment neighbor's thumping stereo all night.

Of course, it is unrealistic to assume you can turn every bedroom into a cocoon that blocks out all light, sound, and activity. You can't stop the train, and you probably won't move just because of the airport (though noisy neighbors might be reason to break a lease). A number of distractions are beyond your control, but for the sake of a good night's sleep, you can eliminate quite a few sleep-inhibiting factors.

You might not realize that some of the following environmental stresses keep you awake. For example, consider the hard-working executive who thinks checking e-mail on his laptop while propped up on his pillow in bed is a way to get ahead of tomorrow's work. Bringing work to bed introduces into the bedroom the same behaviors, feelings, and stresses one might feel in the office. Turn off your e-mail well before bedtime, and don't grade papers, read reports, review presentations, or double-check the financials while curled up under the sheets. Save this work for the morning, or keep it in an office or another room. Separate work and sleep. If you find yourself mentally activated and worrying in bed, set aside some time in the late afternoon or early evening to review tomorrow's to-do list.

Similarly, some nonsleepers watch television as they doze off, justifying it by claiming that the "white noise" calms them. This might be true. But the sounds are also jarring and can disrupt sleep-stage transitions and overall sleep. Eating in bed is also a bad habit that insomniacs should break. Even a bedroom clock can keep you from sleeping, as in Ann's obsession with counting the minutes until her alarm sounded. This is common. If you notice that you worry about the time, try sleeping with your alarm clock facing the other direction. Sleeping without time pressure is easier than playing the time game.

Practicing good sleep hygiene

- Sleep only when you are drowsy.
- If you cannot fall or stay asleep, leave your bedroom and read or engage in a relaxing activity in another room.
- Do not allow yourself to fall asleep outside the bedroom; return to the bed to rest.
- Maintain regular bed and wake times.
- Use your bedroom only for sleep and intimate relations.
- Avoid napping during the day. (If you're extremely exhausted, limit naps to less than one hour, no later than 3 p.m.)
- Avoid caffeine within four to six hours of bedtime.

- Avoid nicotine close to bedtime and during the night.

- Do not drink alcoholic beverages within four to six hours of bedtime.

- Avoid large meals; settle for a small snack before bedtime.

- Avoid strenuous exercise within a few hours of going to sleep.

- Minimize light, noise, and extreme temperatures in the bedroom.

Medical and Psychiatric Disorders Associated with Insomnia

A variety of medical and psychiatric conditions and their treatment can cause insomnia. Insomnia due to psychosocial stressors, medications, psychiatric and medical disorders, and drug or substance abuse is referred to as secondary insomnia.

Here is a list of disorders and conditions that can trigger a secondary insomnia diagnosis:

Psychiatric disorders
Mood disorders: Depression, bipolar disorder, dysthymia
Anxiety disorders: Generalized anxiety disorder, panic disorder, post-traumatic stress disorder
Psychotic disorders: Paranoia, schizophrenia, delusional disorder

Medical disorders
Cardiovascular: Angina, heart failure
Respiratory: Chronic obstructive pulmonary disease, asthma
Neurologic: Alzheimer's disease, Parkinson's disease
Rheumatic: Fibromyalgia, chronic fatigue syndrome, osteoarthritis
Gastrointestinal: Gastroesophageal reflux disease, irritable bowel syndrome
Sleep: Restless legs syndrome, sleep apnea, circadian rhythm disorders

Drug and substance abuse
Alcohol • Tobacco • Recreational drugs • Caffeine

Prescription medications
Beta blockers • Steroids • Levodopa • Stimulants
Thyroid hormone

Acute insomnia

Also referred to as adjustment insomnia, this short-term insomnia is the most common sleep problem. It occurs when a situational stress temporarily disrupts sleep. Transient insomnia can progress into permanent insomnia if sleeplessness persists for more than a few nights and the person cannot break the cycle.

Chronic insomnia

In long-term insomnias, difficulty falling asleep or staying asleep occurs more than a few nights per week for a period of at least six months. More than 70 million Americans complain of insomnia, according to the National Institutes of Health, and being a worrywart isn't the only reason diagnosed individuals stay awake all night. This is why visiting a physician or sleep disorders specialist is especially important. Through the sleep and medical history, sleep questionnaires, and a polysomnogram in select cases, insomniacs can determine whether there are underlying causes for their problem (such as sleep apnea or restless legs syndrome).

Psychophysiological insomnia

First, a person might complain of losing sleep for a few nights. Then the problem escalates into a pattern. Lost sleep intrudes on the person's lifestyle, affecting mood, motivation, performance, and energy level.

Ann is a classic case of psychophysiological insomnia.

She reacted to stress by not sleeping. Her pattern evolved into a lifestyle of losing sleep, and the fatigue further affected her mood and outlook. Soon, bedtime was a greater stress than the emotional tension in her life, and sleeping became an impossible feat – something she feared each night.

Individuals with psychophysiological insomnia might deny stressful events or feelings of depression and anxiety. They blame "insomnia" for their lack of sleep, rather than events in their lives. Insomnia becomes learned, and a vicious cycle develops. The hallmark of psychophysiological insomnia is a person's focus and near obsession with the sleep problem. This attention contributes to sleep loss.

Fifteen percent of all people seen in sleep centers are diagnosed with psychophysiological insomnia, which affects 1 to 2 percent of adults. Onset for psychophysiological insomnia generally occurs in midlife or surrounding a major life stressor (job loss, medical problem, death in family, divorce), and the problem is more frequent in women. It gradually escalates until patients seek treatment.

Note: A psychophysiological insomnia diagnosis is not made in patients diagnosed with anxiety syndromes, phobias, obsessive-compulsive neurosis, major depression, or other psychopathologies. Sleep problems associated with these psychiatric disorders should be treated as part of the psychiatric disorder.

The polysomnogram

Insomnia is usually diagnosed based on the sleep history, and most patients do not require a polysomnogram. Laboratory testing should be considered in patients with insomnia who also have symptoms of sleep apnea or periodic limb movement disorder, and those with typical symptoms who fail to improve with standard treatment. A polysomnogram of a patient diagnosed with psychophysiological insomnia may show prolonged time taken to fall asleep (sleep latency), an increase in stage 1 sleep, and a decrease in stages 3 and 4 sleep (delta or deep sleep), along with frequent arousals. However, sometimes these patients sleep better in the laboratory or a hotel or friend's house than at home, resulting in a "reverse first-night effect." (First-night effect is when the quality of sleep is impaired because of unfamiliar or uncomfortable surroundings. Patients will display more light sleep, less delta sleep and REM sleep, and more arousals and awakenings.)

Behavioral therapy

Improving sleep hygiene is the first step toward establishing a regimen that will promote sound sleep. But patients like Ann also benefit from cognitive behavior therapy. CBT is a broad term applied to a variety of techniques used to treat insomnia and other disorders. The goal is to empower patients and help them gain control over sleep through education. CBT helps correct thought patterns and behaviors that can cause or worsen insomnia, and the approach is not only effective, but its benefits outlast over-the-counter and prescription treatments.

CBT is structured and focused treatment, and patients must play an active role to realize its benefits. A typical session may last forty to sixty minutes, and is usually conducted by a psychologist. The course of treatment varies from six to ten sessions, depending on the intensity of the problem and the patient's progress.

Some of the benefits of CBT include:

- Increase in total sleep time
- Improved sleep efficiency
- Decrease in sleep latency (time it takes to fall asleep)
- Decrease in awakenings during the night

Following are various CBT practices used to correct problematic sleep patterns and reestablish positive thinking about sleep:

1. **Sleep restriction:** Most insomniacs stay in bed too long, frustrated and unable to fall asleep. Sleep restriction allows patients to spend only as much time in bed as they report sleeping (but no less than four hours). When sleep efficiency improves to 85 percent, time in bed is increased in thirty-minute increments.

2. **Relaxation training:** Meditation, progressive relaxation, self-hypnosis, and other techniques that calm the body can help a patient slow down and prepare for sleep.

3. **Stimulus control:** Retraining a patient to see the bedroom as a relaxing place means using the room only for sleep. If a patient is not sleeping, he or she must get out of bed and move to another room. Frustration associates this space with stress, thereby worsening insomnia. The idea is to make this room as peaceful as possible to promote sound sleep.

4. **Biofeedback:** Relaxation is the key. Biofeedback trains a patient to improve health by developing a greater awareness and control over stress and anxiety. Stress and anxiety levels are measured through electrodes placed on the scalp, forehead, chest, abdomen, and fingertip. EEG activity is recorded as the therapist assists the patient in relaxing. This lowers EEG frequencies that facilitate sleep. In respiratory biofeedback, sensors measure respiratory rate, rhythm, and volume. The patient sees and hears breathing patterns during anxiety. A therapist shows the patient how to modify breathing during stressful times.

When sleeping pills help

Ann's physician advised that she continue her sleeping-pill prescription, but taper off usage over a period of six months. A number of sleeping pills are on the market today, and some newer formulas are less addictive and shorter acting than older drugs like valium, preventing patients from feeling a "hangover" or drowsy feeling in the morning that persists hours after awakening.

While sleeping pills can be used to break a bout of insomnia, get on track to improve sleep patterns, and achieve sounder sleep for a period of time, these medications should be used only as a temporary relief. Doctors can prescribe short- or long-acting drugs, depending on when a patient loses sleep. If falling asleep is the problem, short-acting drugs will facilitate sleep and prevent drowsy mornings. If maintaining sleep in the middle of the night is a concern, long-acting drugs provide relief. You should consult a doctor before using these or any type of sleep aid.

Besides prescription sleeping pills, drugstores offer an array of over-the-counter "solutions," though many insomniacs find these ineffective. These drugs include sedating antihistamines.

Many insomniacs rely on sleeping pills as a crutch; they can't sleep without them because they mentally need the drugs. Without them, they worry that they will stay awake all night. (Remember Ann's anxiety when her doctor changed her sleeping-pill prescription. She worried that it would not work as well as her old standby.)

Sleeping pills are not a permanent solution, but they can help in the short term, particularly for patients with acute insomnia related to a sudden, unexpected life stressor and in other situations including jet lag and shift-work schedule changes.

Benzodiazepine hypnotics

Prior to the last several years, these were the drugs of choice to treat insomnia because they were thought to be a safe alternative to barbiturates. Benzodiazepine use is associated with developing tolerance to the drug, dependence, and withdrawal. Use of these drugs to treat insomnia has declined in recent years with the introduction of safer alternatives.

Non-benzodiazepine hypnotics

First introduced to the U.S. market in 1992, non-benzodiazepine hypnotics are an alternative to traditional benzodiazepines and are just as effective. Patients who take non-benzos for insomnia notice decreased incidence of amnesia, daytime sleepiness, respiratory depression, orthostatic hypotension (feeling dizzy when standing or walking), and falls.

Ann's outcome

Ann was evaluated by a sleep specialist and a psychologist with expertise in treating insomnia. She was asked to keep a sleep log to determine the regularity of her sleep-wake cycle. The specialist also instructed her to eliminate caffeine and set aside time each day to plan the next day.

The sleep logs proved very useful, as Ann was spending many hours in bed awake, tossing and turning, which sparked frustration and fed her negative attitude about getting sleep. Her psychologist told her about the twenty-minute toss-and-turn rule and instructed her to get out of bed if she'd been lying awake for twenty minutes or longer. Ann also learned how to use progressive muscle relaxation to clear her mind and distract her from negative sleep thoughts.

Ann's sleeping pill was continued initially. She returned to the psychologist for monthly visits to monitor progress and learn new behavioral strategies. Eventually, she was able to do without her sleeping pill (although she keeps it in the medicine cabinet in the event of an emergency).

People with psychophysiological insomnia usually improve with treatment but rarely sleep as well as they recall sleeping in years past. Ann's motivation and persistence with treatment paid off. But in times of stress, or if she neglected to use the techniques in cognitive behavioral therapy, her sleep quality would quickly revert to sleepless nights.

The Following Prescription Sleep Aids Are Prescribed To Treat Insomnia:

Zolpidem (Ambien): Used for short-term treatment of insomnia. Found to decrease sleep latency and increase duration of sleep. Because of its rapid onset and short duration of action, it is best for sleep-onset insomnia, although a controlled-release form became available in the U.S. last year.

Zaleplon (Sonata): Ultra-short half-life of one hour, which means it has no hangover effect. It is used for short-term treatment of insomnia. Increases total sleep time and decreases awakenings. Best for sleep-onset insomnia; those with middle-of-the-night insomnia can take an extra dose because of its short duration of action.

Eszopiclone (Lunesta): The only hypnotic medication to date approved for long-term use. Decreases sleep latency and wake time after sleep onset; increases sleep efficiency. It has a longer half-life (five to six hours), so it should be used when patients expect to spend at least eight hours in bed. Effective for sleep-onset insomnia and sleep maintenance.

Rozeram: Approved in July 2005 for sleep-onset insomnia, it is the first prescription insomnia medication that targets the normal sleep-wake cycle. It is a melatonin agonist and is the only drug that does not act by depressing the central nervous system. It is also the first insomnia drug that does not have abuse potential.

Note: Dosage adjustments are usually required in seniors and people with liver impairment. All drugs require a prescription from a physician. You should consult a sleep disorders specialist if you detect symptoms of insomnia.

See Appendix 2 for most commonly used sleep aids at drugstore.com.

Chapter 9
Sleep Terrors

> *Sleep is when all the unsorted stuff comes flying out as from a dustbin upset in a high wind.*
>
> *– William Golding*

Sleep terrors *are characterized by a sudden arousal from slow wave sleep. The sleeper will scream, cry, sit up, sweat, have a rapid heartbeat, and display a look of fear. Patients most often do not remember these episodes, which occur during sleep stages 3 and 4.*

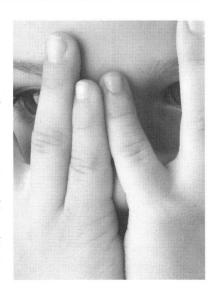

Caleb's blood-curdling scream jarred his mother from a deep sleep. She scurried down the hall and opened her 7-year-old son's bedroom door to find him sitting straight up in his bed – eyes wide open, breathing like he'd been playing tag, rocking back and forth, agitated while he mumbled incoherently.

"Caleb, wake up! It's okay – I'm here."

Caleb looked through his mother as though she were a ghost. The eerie disconnect worried Sandy. She held Caleb's trembling body close to her while he cried, and she smoothed his crop of bed-tousled hair. Caleb carried on for at least five minutes. She thought surely after tucking him into bed more than an hour ago that he would sleep through the night this time.

Caleb's episodes are happening more frequently. The previous week, he woke up almost every night – about an hour after going to bed. Sandy is worried. Caleb never remembers the horrible incidents that scare him into a panic each night. Sometimes he is aggressive, thrashing and protesting when Sandy tries to shake him out of his frightened stupor. Just recently, he ran out of the bedroom, down the stairs, and toward the front door. Fortunately, it was locked. Despite all her efforts, Sandy's attempts to calm him down are futile.

Sandy called Caleb's pediatrician to discuss the behavior, and both agreed that Caleb is not simply having recurring bad dreams. Caleb's behavior worries the doctor. The young boy could accidentally hurt himself or someone else. The doctor suggested that Caleb and his mother see a sleep specialist.

Caleb's sleep assessment

Sleep snapshot

Caleb's bedtime is between 8:30 and 9 p.m., and he slept soundly through the night before his incidents began a few months ago. His frightening episodes usually occur in cycles, eventually increasing in frequency to every night for a week. He does not display excessive daytime sleepiness or difficulty falling back asleep after one of his episodes. In general, Caleb is a healthy boy, and his medical records show no medical or psychological concerns.

The sleep specialist recommended an overnight sleep study for Caleb, but told Sandy that he suspected sleep terrors. A polysomnogram might help the physician to differentiate sleep terrors from nocturnal seizures, a condition also characterized by recurrent episodes of abnormal behaviors in sleep. The physician wanted to rule out disorders known to aggravate sleep terrors, such as sleep apnea since Sandy reported that Caleb occasionally snores. Because Caleb is quite young, his mother was asked to accompany him to the lab and stay with him during the study.

The technologists applied electrodes to Caleb's scalp and attached other sensors to record Caleb's breathing, heart rate, oxygen level, and body movements while he slept. Prior to the study, his mother signed a consent form for Caleb to be videotaped. (Video is now routine during overnight sleep studies. It helps the physician interpret the study by correlating brain and breathing signals with movements and behaviors in sleep.)

Not surprisingly, the young boy did not have any abnormal activity through the night, other than some difficulty in falling asleep due to the sensors and the strange environment. The "negative polysomnogram" didn't confirm the suspected diagnosis, but it did rule out other sleep disorders, such as periodic limb movements and apnea. Also, the physician was less concerned about epileptic seizures. Negative polysomnograms in this setting are not uncommon, the physician explained to Caleb's mother. The best alternative for Caleb was for his mother to videotape him sleeping at home in his own bed.

Sometimes, especially in cases like Caleb's where video is a critical factor for diagnosis, conducting a "study" at home is just as effective as checking into a lab. Your doctor will advise if this is a viable option. Sandy captured several of Caleb's episodes on tape, and the physician observed the recordings. The similarity of one event to another, time of occurrence from the time Caleb went to bed, and his facial expressions and vocalization helped Caleb's physician make a diagnosis.

The diagnosis

After reviewing the videotapes, the sleep specialist diagnosed Caleb with sleep terrors. His behavior aligned with the disorder's symptoms: abrupt arousal from deep sleep, screaming, crying, pallor, panic, and lack of response to wake-up attempts.

All about sleep terrors

Sleep terrors are a mysterious sleep disorder in the parasomnia category in which patients experience an incomplete arousal from deep sleep. The patient appears to be aware but is usually non-responsive to the environment. Sleep terrors tend to happen in cycles; a person may experience one episode in his or her entire life or recurrent episodes as often as every night.

Many individuals who suffer from sleep terrors are misdiagnosed. Children are often told, "It's just a nightmare, don't worry." Adults are misdiagnosed with post-traumatic stress disorder or nocturnal panic disorder, or often don't even report the unusual behavior to their doctors at all. It is important to understand the distinction among these disorders and to note that night terrors are a fright-ening, confusing experience for sleepers and observers alike. You can't shake a person out of a sleep terror, and the frightened sleeper will not respond to your voice no matter how loud. The best thing to do is to comfort with a hug and assure the person in a soothing tone that everything will be okay. (Of course, this might not be possible if the person is thrashing or violent, which is more common in adults.) However, attempts to restrain the sleeper may provoke more aggressive responses.

An overnight sleep study can help determine which stage of sleep the patient is in when the terror occurs. If increased brain activity is detected during slow wave sleep (stages 3 and 4), then a diagnosis of sleep terrors is likely.

What causes sleep terrors?

During the third and fourth stages of non-REM sleep, the brain is in its deepest state – a state in which the mind and body rejuvenate. Arousing from deep sleep is not the norm. Unlike in REM sleep, when the body is essentially paralyzed, the body reacts when brain activity transitions into sleep. This usually occurs within the first hour after sleep onset. The person is still sleeping but able to act out. Bedwetting, sleeptalking, and sleepwalking also occur during stages 3 and 4.

People who have sleep terrors usually do not remember the incidents. Rarely, the patient may recall portions of a vivid dream that was frightening in nature. In fact, when an observer watches a child have a sleep terror, the child looks truly frightened. During the terror, patients' eyes may open, pupils dilate, and they may sit up in bed abruptly and breathe heavily. Heart rate during these incidents can pump up to 170 beats per minute, far exceeding the normal, resting heart rate. The episode might last five to twenty minutes, during which time the person might scream out, babble incoherently, thrash, and in some cases, bolt out of bed and run out of the room. (This is more common in adults.)

For this reason, sleep terrors are potentially dangerous. Patients who suffer from them can injure themselves unknowingly. Patients are difficult to arouse during sleep terrors, and may be confused or disoriented upon awakening. Because the majority of stages 3 and 4 occur in the first third of the sleep period, episodes also tend to occur during this time.

When disturbed sleepers do remember sleep terror incidents, they often report seeing animals or people – quite a few see snakes and spiders. Science cannot explain this imagery.

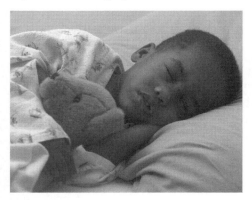

Who gets sleep terrors?

Sleep terrors are most common in children ages 3 to 12, and they tend to resolve during adolescence. Up to 6 percent of children may experience sleep terrors. A much smaller population of adults experience this disorder (closer to 2 percent). Incidents are most common in adults ages 20 to 30. Few individuals over age 65 experience sleep terrors. Family history may play a strong role in whether your child will experience these episodes.

Sleep terrors often occur or increase in frequency during times of stress or exhaustion. For example, a child going through a transition in school is more likely to experience an episode. Also, a child who had an exhausting day is more prone to a sleep terror come bedtime.

Nightmare or sleep terror?

One key differentiation between a sleep terror and a nightmare is the time of the attack. Because sleep terrors occur during deep sleep, episodes take place in the first part of the night, usually an hour or two after bedtime. On the other hand, a nightmare, which usually occurs during rapid eye movement sleep, will occur toward the end of the night. However, there are exceptions to this rule.

Another distinction is whether you can wake up a person during the episode. During a sleep terror, a person's eyes may open, but he or she will see right through you. In fact, the sleeper has no idea you are present and will not respond to your voice or touch.

On the other hand, if the incident is a nightmare, the person's eyes also may open and he or she may scream. But the frightened individual usually wakes up because of the dream and will respond to comforting.

Nightmares vs. Sleep Terrors

Not sure if your child – or spouse – is waking up frightened from a sleep terror or nightmare? Here is the difference:

Sleep Terror	Nightmare
Occurs in first third of night	Occurs during REM sleep (usually last third of night)
Will not respond to touch	Will respond to touch and comforting sound, or attempts to comfort
Confused after episode; doesn't remember episode	Is fully awake after episode; often recalls dreams

How to get a good night's sleep

Do not try to yell, coax, or shake a child out of a sleep terror. During this deep sleep stage, the child is having an incomplete arousal; this means he or she is still technically asleep, yet able to move and appears awake. Your child likely will not remember the incident, so pressing for information or explanations the next morning will only lead to frustration. Instead, if you notice that sleep terrors are a pattern, stand by the bedroom door and observe your child. Call your pediatrician and explain the behavior.

On the other hand, young children will unknowingly appreciate a hug and comforting touch. Though they will probably not respond to comforting actions, holding a child is a natural and healthy reaction to sleep terrors. Some believe that by gently waking up your child as he or she is falling asleep, you can disrupt the sleep patterns that could be sparking sleep terrors. However, this could also cause your child to lose more sleep and not affect behavior as he or she progresses into deeper sleep stages.

Your physician might recommend certain medications to calm these episodes. These are used as a temporary solution until the patient resolves behavior. Caleb was prescribed imipramine, which also is used to treat bedwetting. Other possible medications include diazepam and amitryptiline. Medications are generally reserved for severe cases – when episodes occur frequently or are particularly disruptive to others in the household. Your doctor will indicate whether these medications are appropriate.

Because exhaustion and stress can spur sleep terrors, ensure that your child gets enough rest. If your child usually takes a nap, make sure there is time for this important period of rest. If bedtimes are getting later and wake-up calls earlier, adjust sleep schedules so your child won't wear out during the day. Normal routines foster healthy sleep habits, and your child's activities during the day will have an impact on his or her ability to sleep soundly.

Caleb's outcome

Caleb was treated with imipramine, which significantly reduced the frequency and severity of episodes. After eighteen months of treatment, his physician gradually withdrew the medication and he remained spell-free.

Chapter 10

Rapid Eye Movement (REM) Behavior Disorder

If you want your spouse to listen and pay strict attention to every word you say, talk in your sleep.

– *Anonymous*

Don't kill the dream – execute it.

– *Anonymous*

REM behavior disorder *occurs when the physical paralysis characteristic of REM sleep is incomplete or absent. This condition allows individuals to act out their dreams.*

Janet and Tom never pick fights with one another. Their happy, fifteen-year marriage has been punctuated by only a few real arguments. Tom simply isn't a confrontational person, and Janet would rather compromise than bicker. Lately, Tom's behavior has shifted – but only while he sleeps.

Janet regularly wakes up to a kicking, thrashing, seemingly angry Tom. He flails his arms, slamming his fist on the mattress like a gavel while he speaks loudly, often swearing. Tom never talked like that. He always kept his cool, no matter how angry he was.

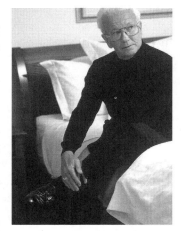

Tom doesn't remember these confrontations when he wakes up, no matter how violent or disturbing they are. He has always had vivid dreams and, though he admits he sometimes can't separate reveries from reality, the actual content of his discussions always surprise him. Janet worries he will hurt himself – or her. She connects his vulgar and angry language to past arguments with subordinates at work. Tom, 62, was diagnosed with Parkinson's disease eight years ago and retired four years later.

Lately, he is more forgetful and struggles to concentrate. Mostly, he complains that his restless nights take a toll on his energy level. He wakes up four to six times each night and does not fall back asleep easily. He snores, suffers from daytime sleepiness, and can't restrain his nocturnal activities. What's more, his condition only seems to get worse. Recently, he gave Janet a black eye during a nocturnal struggle.

Tom's sleep assessment

Sleep snapshot

Tom turns in at 9 p.m. and wakes up at 5 a.m. He says six hours of sleep is sufficient, but he generally only gets four to five hours of rest each night, interrupted by frequent awakenings.

Excessive daytime sleepiness

Though Tom wakes up refreshed in the morning, he always takes early evening naps. By then, his sleepless night catches up with him, and he feels much better if he can capture ten to twenty minutes of shut-eye before dinner. Tom denies excessive daytime sleepiness, but the physician scored Tom's Epworth Sleepiness Scale at 15 out of 24 – a significantly higher rating than normal.

Parasomnias

Tom's behavior is characteristic of a parasomnia, a disorder in which the patient experiences unusual sleep behavior, often without recollection. Some parasomnia behaviors include sleepwalking, sleeptalking, and sleep-related eating. These disorders usually arise from NREM sleep. During these periods of apparent wakefulness, they engage in unusual behavior.

Tom acts out his dreams. His episodes almost always occur in the wee morning hours, and he sometimes recalls vivid frightening dreams where he is threatened or chased. These symptoms suggest there may be a disconnect in REM sleep. During this stage, the body is paralyzed, but the mind is active. Normal sleepers' still bodies aren't in sync with their stimulated brains, but this prevents them from acting out dreams. In Tom's case, his body is not paralyzed in REM sleep as it should be, leading to the ability to move in response to threatening dreams.

The diagnosis

Tom displays symptoms of REM behavior disorder (RBD), when paralysis during REM is cut short or not present at all. He dreams wildly and has the ability to act out each scene. Parkinson's disease is known to be associated with RBD. In fact,

80 percent of patients with this neurodegenerative disorder suffer from a primary sleep disorder. Tom's sleepwalking and violent bedtime behavior have worsened since he was diagnosed with Parkinson's disease, but in retrospect, Janet remembers him having occasional screaming spells years before the Parkinson's set in.

RBD was an obvious conclusion after conducting a sleep interview. The physician ordered an overnight polysomnogram and MSLT with expanded EMG and EEG sensors to collect more detailed brain-wave and muscle activity data. Additional sensors help confirm an RBD diagnosis by analyzing the level of muscle activity during REM sleep. Also, expanded information is critical to ruling out the multitude of other sleep disorders known to affect Parkinson's patients, including restless legs syndrome, periodic limb movement disorder, sleep apnea, and daytime sleepiness spurred by medications.

All about REM behavior disorder

Some of the most unusual sleep stories come from individuals with REM behavior disorder. Take Edward, who broke his leg "saving himself" by jumping out a window to escape from a fire he dreamed. Or consider the patient whose wife locked him into a bedroom each night because his behavior was so disturbing and violent. Then there's the husband who dreamed he was being chased and ran out the front door. And how about the restless sleeper and otherwise kind young man who took a swing at his mate when he thought he was in the middle of a standoff?

Most RBD patients are, in fact, men. A typical profile is a male over age 60 who might demonstrate other brain disorders. RBD is not a psychiatric disorder, but it is a potentially dangerous neurological condition that can be treated.

RBD is in the REM parasomnia category. There are a dozen parasomnias, and they can occur in both REM and NREM sleep stages. Most common are sleeptalking and sleepwalking. RBD takes sleepwalking to a new level. Rather than trolling around like a zombie, these individuals are animated and involved in their dreams.

RBD is differentiated from arousal disorders because it occurs during REM sleep, when the body is supposed to be paralyzed. There is loss of REM sleep atonia – the limp, paralyzed state associated with this sleep stage – which allows those with RBD to move freely, even violently. Kicking, thrashing, and running from bed – usually escaping from someone or something chasing them – are not unusual actions for RBD patients.

These incidents typically occur in the last one-third of the sleep period, when REM sleep predominates. But they can occur as early as ninety minutes after sleep onset during the first REM period. Violent episodes can occur as infrequently as a few times in a lifetime or as frequently as several times over several consecutive nights. Most patients complain of sleep injury but rarely cite sleep disruption, as they usually do not wake up until a family member jerks them back into reality. Once awake, patients often recall their dramatic dreams.

Who gets RBD?

RBD usually surfaces in men 50 or older. The disorder is linked to medical problems, most notably Parkinson's disease and related neurodegenerative disorders associated with dementia, strokes, and narcolepsy. In fact, 30 percent of Parkinson's patients have RBD, and symptoms of RBD may precede other neurological problems by up to ten years. Two-thirds of men who have RBD will eventually develop Parkinsonism. In some instances, a temporary form of RBD can occur during withdrawal from alcohol, sedatives, or some antidepressants.

How do you know you have RBD?

Patients who have the disorder may display one or more of the following symptoms. Ask yourself these questions:

- Do you act out dreams?
- Do you ever thrash, punch, kick, or run away from your bed, and do you recall these incidents?
- Do you recall vivid, threatening dreams after waking?
- Are you tired during the day because of restless nights?
- Does your bed partner complain of violent behavior or does he/she notice activity while you sleep?

Severity

There are several levels of RBD. Mild cases display behavior less than once per month and cause mild discomfort to bed partners. Patients with moderate RBD act out less than once a week and create a physically uncomfortable situation for their bed partners. Patients with severe RBD are violent and cause physical injury to themselves and their bed partners.

The polysomnogram

During REM sleep, patients with RBD will show signs of augmented muscle tone. If awakened during an episode, patients might relay a dream that correlates with their physical activity. Periodic leg movements, arm activity, and otherwise restless behavior are also observed in sleepers diagnosed with RBD.

How to get a good night's sleep

Sleep histories are critical in making an RBD diagnosis. A polysomnogram helps to confirm the diagnosis and rule out other sleep disorders, such as periodic limb movements and sleep apnea. A physician might order other tests, such as brain imaging, to determine whether a patient has associated neurological disorders as well. Typically, RBD can be treated by medications used to suppress REM sleep, which also inhibits physical activity.

RBD and neurodegenerative diseases

We know there is an increased rate of RBD in people with neurodegenerative diseases, but the latest research suggests that RBD could be a sign of other degenerative processes in the central nervous system.

If RBD is one of the earliest stages on the neurodegenerative spectrum, perhaps in the future, physicians could test for RBD and treat patients with medication that may ward off these more debilitating disorders. Researchers are hopeful that medical advances will make earlier identification and treatment possible in years to come.

Tom's outcome

Tom's polysomnogram showed nearly continuous limb (leg and arm) movements in both NREM and REM sleep. During NREM sleep, particularly stages 1 and 2, frequent periodic limb movements caused arousal, leading to excessive fragmentation of sleep. Tom even had periodic leg movements when he was awake at the start of the study. In REM sleep, he showed elevated amounts of muscle tone in his arms and legs, and had a couple of episodes where he vocalized incoherently and flailed his arms, but nothing as dramatic as he has at home.

Tom was placed on clonazepam, a drug in the benzodiazepine class, which is considered a sedative hypnotic. This is the treatment of choice for RBD, and even low doses are able to abolish spells in many cases. This agent is also effective in treating restless legs syndrome and periodic limb movement disorder.

Chapter 11

Circadian Rhythm Sleep Disorders/Delayed Sleep-Phase Syndrome

> *"Dawn: when men of reason go to bed."*
>
> – Ambrose Bierce

Circadian rhythm sleep disorders *occur when normal sleep-wake rhythms are disturbed, many times when an individual's natural sleep-wake schedule does not conform to society's norm. These disorders are due to alterations of the internal body clock or misalignment between the body's internal rhythms and environmental factors.*

Delayed sleep-phase syndrome *is a circadian rhythm disorder most common in adolescents and young adults, whose "night owl" tendencies delay sleep onset – often until 2 a.m. or later. Early wake times result in sleep-deprivation, daytime sleepiness, and impaired work and school performance.*

Andy never was a morning person. He hits his peak at 10 p.m. and can't fall asleep until after 2 a.m., no matter how hard he tries. Even in high school when his mother turned off the television promptly at 10, he would lie in bed wide-awake until well after midnight. She always figured Andy was asleep, and she never understood why he was so groggy at breakfast.

When Andy, now 20, went away to college, the late-night/party weekend schedule jibed with his night-owl tendencies. His freshman year, he turned out the lights at 1 a.m. during the week. But Andy's internal "closing time" on Friday and Saturday nights (and sometimes Thursdays, if Friday classes were canceled) usually neared 3 or 4 a.m. He slept away Saturday and Sunday mornings, waking barely in time for lunch.

Andy chalked up his routine to campus life. When his mom expressed concern, he shrugged, rolled his eyes, and said, "Whatever, Mom."

Now that Andy's a sophomore, he's found he no longer can avoid early classes. He has a 9 a.m. lab two days a week and an 8 a.m. history class the other days.

And he can't seem to adjust his bedtime to get the sleep he needs. He's tried everything: reading, avoiding weekday activities, and even taking over-the-counter sleep aids. Nothing works. Alcohol makes him feel less rested the next day.

Now, Andy's grades are slipping. And his mom, of course, is asking questions.

Andy's sleep assessment

Sleep snapshot

Andy doesn't fall asleep until 1 or 2 a.m. during the week and much later on weekends, but this bedtime is consistent. He can't alter it – he'll only lie in bed awake. He usually sleeps for six hours each night. On weekends when he can sleep in late, he gets a solid eight hours, sometimes ten hours, and feels great when he wakes up. And once Andy falls asleep, he sleeps soundly until morning (or early afternoon). He's sluggish only during the school week when he is forced to rise earlier than he would like.

Medical and family history

Andy's mother finds his behavior a bit unusual. She and her husband sleep soundly, with the exception of some occasional snoring. In fact, she's quite the opposite of Andy, usually waking up cheery and chirping "good morning" to her grouchy son. Neither she nor her husband have been diagnosed or treated for sleep disorders.

Excessive daytime sleepiness

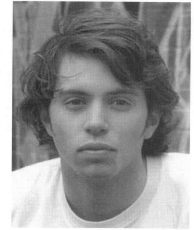

Andy isn't alert in the morning, and he drags through afternoons because he's so tired from waking up for early classes. He rarely has time for naps, as campus life is so busy. But he has been observed snoozing in Chemistry 101 – the professor made him aware of that.

Andy's teachers have pointed out his slipping grades. He's a bright and creative student, but his professors don't see him at his peak; they only know the tired, unmotivated "slacker."

Because Andy struggles to fall asleep at night, his mother questioned whether his delayed sleep onset was a sign of insomnia. Conversely, Andy wondered if he was narcoleptic because he falls asleep during class sometimes, and he's even dozed off while driving long distances.

The diagnosis

Andy's physician requested that he keep a sleep diary for two weeks, recording the following information:

- Bedtime and wake time
- How long it took to fall asleep
- Number of awakenings during the night; length of these awakenings
- Number of times he got out of bed
- Total sleep time
- How he felt when he woke up in the morning
- Number and quality of daytime naps

A tailored test for Andy

Andy maintained a sleep log for two weeks, and the physician noticed an obvious sleep pattern. His sleep was quite different on weekdays versus weekends. He slept soundly for eight to ten hours on weekends, and he always woke refreshed as long as he didn't have to get up early for school. However, his bedtimes and wake times were out-of-sync with what most people consider normal.

The physician ordered an overnight sleep study and MSLT so he could observe Andy's sleep-wake cycle in the lab. Because the physician already understood Andy's sleep patterns, the polysomnogram and MSLT were tailored to meet his habits. That way, the study would produce the best results possible because it would measure Andy's cycles when his body naturally triggered sleep.

What a customized polysomnogram and MSLT uncovered about Andy

The tailored polysomnogram was important for Andy, given his tendency to stay awake at night and sleep in late. In the lab, Andy fell asleep around 3 a.m., which the physician expected. His polysomnogram showed a few arousals during sleep, but no significant apnea episodes or limb movements. Because technologists knew of Andy's natural sleep patterns, they allowed him to sleep much later than the typical 6 a.m. wake-up time so they could record his complete sleep period. He slept for nearly eight hours.

Andy's MSLT started at noon rather than 8 a.m. His sleep latency during the MSLT was twelve minutes, and he did not enter REM sleep. He described his sleep in the lab as "typical" for a weekend.

Andy's results ruled out insomnia and narcolepsy. He did not nap frequently or have any of the other cardinal features of narcolepsy. Also, the physician knew that Andy's sleep onset was delayed during the polysomnogram because his circadian clock was timed so his body wants to sleep much later than the average person. Unlike insomniacs, Andy did not experience frequent arousals or stay awake for long periods of time during the night, nor did he have anxiety about not being able to fall asleep at night. Though he didn't fall asleep until 3 a.m., the delayed onset was typical behavior according to his sleep log.

Based on this information, the physician diagnosed Andy with delayed sleep-phase syndrome.

Tailored Tests

Tailoring sleep lab tests is critical to properly diagnosing many sleep disorders. Consider Andy. If he had not kept a sleep diary or provided a sleep history, the physician would not know that the young man habitually falls asleep at 2 a.m., rarely wakes up, and can sleep soundly for hours if allowed. This kind of information is critical to tailoring the sleep study to diagnose Andy's problem. Daytime tests often begin around 8 a.m. Had Andy been awakened by the technologist to start the daytime test on time, the results might have led to a misdiagnosis. Andy may have appeared to have insomnia or difficulty adjusting to the sleep lab environment. Then, during his MSLT, his sleep latency may have been only minutes, and he might have plunged into REM sleep, which would have suggested narcolepsy.

Neither of these diagnoses would have been accurate for Andy.

All about delayed sleep-phase syndrome

Delayed sleep-phase syndrome (DSPS) often surfaces during adolescent and early-adult years. Patients diagnosed with the disorder have difficulty conforming to society's time schedule and often are perceived as lazy, unmotivated, or poor performers. In fact, people like Andy are productive, alert, and creative later at night. The problem is a conflict between these individuals' circadian rhythms and what is expected or considered the norm.

College life mimics DSPS. Many times, young adults adopt poor sleep hygiene in college and, as a result, develop alternative sleeping patterns. They stay up late, sleep in late, and make up for lost sleep on weekends. Sleeping for eight hours isn't a problem – as long as it's on their schedules.

But when individuals with DSPS enter the "real world," they struggle to wake up for work and often find themselves lying awake at night if they try to force themselves to sleep before their bodies are ready. They often are chronically tardy or perform poorly on the job. You can't force people with DSPS to fall asleep, and you can't shift their circadian rhythm without proper treatment.

Because those diagnosed with DSPS suffer from sleep deprivation, many of them turn to beverages like Mountain Dew, which is the powerhouse of caffeinated drinks, or energy drinks like Red Bull. Or they may take over-the-counter stimulants like No-Doz. To sleep at night, they try sleep aids, which don't work for them. Maybe they go out for a nightcap, which worsens their sleep cycles, perpetuates symptoms, and may even lead to substance abuse.

Symptoms of DSPS

- Sleep onset is later than desired, usually between 1 and 6 a.m., though it occurs at the same time each night

- Wake times in the late morning or early afternoon if undisturbed

- Little or no difficulty staying asleep following sleep onset

- Difficulty waking in the early morning

- Inability to fall asleep earlier

- Daytime sleepiness, resulting in unplanned naps and feeling unrefreshed after waking

- Poor academic performance, falling asleep during classes or being unproductive at work, viewed as lazy or unmotivated, and chronically tardy for morning activities

Treating DSPS

The best ways to treat DSPS are methods that promote earlier sleep and wake-up times. While practicing good sleep hygiene (discussed in Chapter 8) is the first step toward creating a relaxing, sleep-happy environment, there are other ways to adjust circadian rhythm.

Essentially, DSPS patients need to trick their biological clocks into thinking it is time for bed between 10 p.m. and midnight; and they need to promote wakefulness at a "normal" hour like 7 a.m. To do this, a physician might prescribe melatonin or suggest light therapy.

Melatonin

You may have heard of melatonin as a "helper" for jet lag. Melatonin is a hormone normally secreted by the pineal gland in the brain to promote sleep. Melatonin excretion occurs when it is dark; daylight suppresses melatonin. In those with DSPS, melatonin release may be delayed, which explains why they may not feel sleepy until the early morning hours. Melatonin levels can be checked to help confirm the diagnosis, but this is usually done for research purposes. A physician may prescribe a specific dosage of melatonin to jump-start the brain's natural melatonin secretion to be taken several hours before bedtime (6 p.m. is a good starting point for many patients).

Light therapy

Daylight tells the body, "Time to wake up!" Consistent exposure to bright light tends to lead to earlier wake-up times and to advance sleep onset at night. Patients can receive this therapy at home by using a light box, which emits a standard dosage of 10,000 lux (a measurement of illumination). This brightness mirrors natural sunlight. A DSPS sleeper will clip the light to his or her bed, position it at a specified distance from the face, and turn it on in the morning after waking. These lights also can be put on a timer, which is helpful for most DSPS patients who are just as likely to avoid the bright light as they are a buzzing alarm clock. The light will stimulate the brain to wake up even if the patient is lying in bed with eyes closed.

Dosage and timing of light treatment depends on the patient. For some, light exposure beginning at 7 a.m. may gradually advance sleep onset at night by a couple of hours. It's equally important for the person with DPSP to avoid bright light exposure in the evening. Sufferers should minimize brightly lit rooms, computer screens, and other sources of light after 8 p.m.

Andy's outcome

While Andy's case at first sounds like "typical college stuff," he faced a serious sleep deficit that affected his mood and performance in school – and, ultimately, his future. To gradually shift Andy's bedtime to midnight, the physician prescribed melatonin in addition to morning light therapy. Andy found the treatment tedious at first but changed his attitude when his performance improved.

At school, Andy's grades were better, and his attention span during class improved. He no longer dragged himself out of bed to get to class and stopped dozing in sedentary situations. Andy maintained the same treatment on weekends to develop a consistent schedule. While he accepted that DSPS is a lifelong condition, he felt at ease knowing that treatment would help him achieve his goals and keep up with his friends and colleagues.

Other circadian rhythm disorders

DSPS is the most common circadian rhythm disorder among adolescents and young adults, but other populations experience sleep deprivation from a skewed body clock. Do your sleep patterns match society's ideas of appropriate bedtimes and wake-up calls? Here are a few disorders that occur when lifestyle plays with sleep cycles:

Advanced sleep-phase syndrome

The opposite of DSPS, ASPS is most common in mature adults, who naturally want to go to bed sooner. A senior may fall asleep at 6 p.m. and wake up at 2 a.m. This pattern can disrupt social activities during the day because the individual is fatigued from such an uncommonly early wake-up time.

Light therapy can be used for patients with ASPS. However, in contrast to DSPS, the treatment is administered in the evening to delay sleep onset. It is important to rule out depression, which is another cause of early morning awakening.

Shift work sleep disorder

If you go to sleep at 7 a.m. and wake up at 3 p.m. to prepare for your night shift, your body won't reverse back into "normal" gear when you have a weekend off to spend with 9-to-5'ers. Such drastic switches in bed and wake times take a toll on the body and the brain. While you attempt to shift your circadian clock, you live in a world where social and physical activities are designed for a different schedule. Those who suffer from shift work sleep disorder often feel in disarray.

Light exposure can help reset circadian clocks. It often is used in occupational settings to promote wakefulness outside of normal business hours. On the other hand, keeping the room dim at bedtime will help promote sleep when the worker needs it. Workers should establish an environment free of distraction so they can sleep during the day.

Recently, Provigil received FDA approval for daytime sleepiness in shift workers. Shift workers with daytime sleepiness, insomnia, or impaired performance should consult their physician to rule out sleep disorders such as sleep apnea and periodic limb movements that may be adding insult to injury.

Jet lag disorder

Jet lag occurs when insomnia or daytime sleepiness develop due to transmeridian jet travel across at least two time zones. Impaired functioning and physical symptoms like gastrointestinal upset are often present. Eastward travel that requires advancing sleep onset is more difficult to adjust to than westward travel, when sleep onset is delayed.

Melatonin is often used to promote sleep so individuals with jet lag can reset their circadian clocks. It is important for travelers to conform to the time zone of their destination and to avoid sleeping before it is dark. This is the best way to reestablish sleeping patterns and avoid severe daytime sleepiness.

Chapter 12
Sleep in Special Populations

*People who say they sleep like a baby
usually don't have one.*

— Leo J. Burke

Sleeping habits start in the crib and change as we age. Usually, parents establish the foundation for healthy habits that promote sleep. They introduce us to bedtime rituals, which might include a favorite storybook, a glass of warm milk, a nightlight, and the assurance that Mom and Dad are not far away.

As we grow older, our lifestyles evolve into a complicated web of school, friends, hobbies, relationships, careers, and emotional trials that inevitably interfere with our sleeping patterns. Illness, medications, and psychiatric problems can cloud our dreams and turn a good night into a nightmare. For every stage of life, there are obstacles we face in pursuit of sound sleep.

How can we establish and maintain habits that will prepare us to obtain quality sleep throughout life? And, in populations most vulnerable to change – particularly children and older adults – what are some signs of potential sleep disorders?

We know that sleep is critical to health at every age. We also know that children and older adults are more prone to certain sleep disorders, and these special populations also experience "normal" body functions that can be confused with disorders. In this chapter, we will identify:

- Ways to understand why sleep is so important for children and seniors

- What symptoms are normal signs of aging

- Symptoms that could indicate a sleep disorder

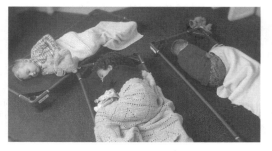

Children and sleep

Children ages 5 to 12 need ten to eleven hours of sleep each night.

When sleep suffers, children:

- Forget what they learned in school
- Are grumpy and ornery
- Have difficulty concentrating on games or playing sports
- Are less patient with their siblings and friends
- Will "turn off" requests from teachers and parents, or have a tough time listening in general

On the other hand, children who sleep well at night and whose parents establish and enforce bedtime rituals are more attentive, creative, and healthy. But sound sleep starts well before a child can communicate feelings of fatigue, hunger, or fear.

Sleeping babies (sometimes) lie

When an infant fusses, a parent's natural reaction is to run to the crib to comfort and calm the little one. Parents are especially sensitive to the sounds of their

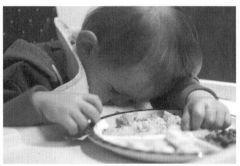

upset children. But when this habit occurs every hour, every night, parents must take measures to improve sleep quality for the whole family.

Certain medical conditions, such as colic, might explain why your infant is agitated at night. Describe your child's sleeping patterns to your pediatrician, who can provide advice on how many hours your baby should sleep each night and offer guidance for helping your child establish nighttime sleep habits. Usually, problems are a matter of learned behavior and can be cleared up with a little advice from your doctor or other parents.

Remember, parents play the primary role in promoting sound sleep for their children. Just as we learn how to tie our shoes and ride a bike, we must learn how to sleep through the night. This is possible only when parents set boundaries.

Teaching bedtime

Sleep-onset disorder

I can hear the rustling in the crib and first hiccups of a night tantrum through the baby monitor before Emma starts a fit. I know I shouldn't go to her every time she cries, but I can't stand to hear her so unhappy. If I hold her and pace the nursery, she is usually asleep on my shoulder in ten minutes. The only problem is that this has become a routine every two hours.

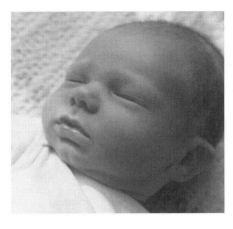

Every person wakes up for short periods of time during the night; we usually do not remember these awakenings because they are so brief. But children can respond differently to nighttime arousals. They might feel insecure or frightened, and they express these emotions by crying.

Parents naturally want to comfort their baby. This becomes a problem when the child associates falling asleep with being held, walked around the room, rocked, or driven around the block. Rather than learning to fall asleep on her own, the baby requires a parent's touch. Without this contact, the child experiences great difficulty falling back asleep.

To correct the problem, you must teach the baby to fall asleep without your help. If you typically "rescue" your child several times each night, a gradual approach is best. First, make sure there is something in the room to comfort your baby when you are not there. A CD player attached to the crib that can play lullabies or a white noise machine often does the trick. The point is to help your child associate sleep onset with something other than you.

When your baby cries at night, avoid immediate response. This can be more difficult for the parent than for the child, but by returning to the child's room seconds after fussing begins, you will re-teach the association you are trying to break. Here is a technique that might assist you over a six-month period in teaching your child to fall asleep without your presence.

First, tuck your child in and say goodnight. (Remember that infants should always be put to bed on their backs; tummy-sleeping is associated with Sudden Infant Death Syndrome or SIDS.) Leave the room, and be sure to allow a little light to enter the nursery. If your child is still crying after a couple of minutes, return to the room and comfort her with words or touching her back to show safety and comfort. If your child continues to cry, wait longer to return to the room, still resisting the temptation to pick up or hold her. After a few nights, parents usually see improvement.

Curbing nighttime appetites

Excessive nighttime feeding can cause parents and children to lose sleep. Overfeeding translates to several times during the night for infants and even one nightly feeding for babies 6 to 11 months old. (Talk to your pediatrician for more specific guidelines, as each child has different needs.) Similar to sleep onset association, if parents feed children several times during the night, they might actually learn to be hungry when they are not.

Not sure if your baby craves the bottle too much during the night? Check his diaper. If it is soaked when the child wakes during the night, he could be eat-

ing too much. If this is the case, gradually reduce the number of nighttime feedings. You can start by decreasing the quantity in the bottle or by waiting two hours between feedings the first night and gradually increasing times between feedings.

Set limits

Toddlers can invent creative reasons why parents should extend bedtime by reading just one more book or refilling a juice glass. A child may stall bedtime with special requests for hugs, tissues, or an urgent need to ask a parent an important question. *Will you turn the lights on? I'm scared when the door is closed. Can I sleep with you tonight? But I'm not tired …*

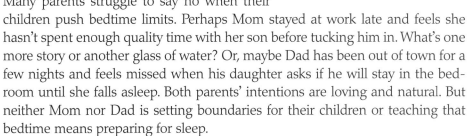

Many parents struggle to say no when their children push bedtime limits. Perhaps Mom stayed at work late and feels she hasn't spent enough quality time with her son before tucking him in. What's one more story or another glass of water? Or, maybe Dad has been out of town for a few nights and feels missed when his daughter asks if he will stay in the bedroom until she falls asleep. Both parents' intentions are loving and natural. But neither Mom nor Dad is setting boundaries for their children or teaching that bedtime means preparing for sleep.

Quality time before bed is an important part of a nighttime ritual. Establish a routine with your children so you can spend quality time together – with limits.

The good sleep hygiene that is essential for promoting sound sleep in adults is just as important for children and perhaps more so, as they are learning how to fall asleep on their own.

Bedtime ritual

Set a bedtime. If children know that 8 p.m. is when they should be under the covers – no exceptions for babysitters or caregivers – they will not protest when a parent starts the bedtime process.

Brush teeth, get ready for bed. Even establishing basic habits such as these will help set a routine for children so they associate a sequence of events with sleep.

Read a story. Winding down the evening with a storybook is a good way for parents to spend quality time before bed. This routine also signals to children that it is "quiet time." Just don't let one story turn into a book series. If children know that Mom reads one book, or each parent reads one story, they will not bargain for a later bedtime.

Say goodnight. These words are a conclusion to the day – activities are over, time for bed. This verbal trigger lets children know that they must close their eyes and go to sleep.

Leave the room. You may turn on a nightlight or keep a door cracked open if these conditions make your child feel more secure.

Do not:

- Substitute a television program for personal interaction
- Allow your child to fall asleep with a bottle or while being rocked or held
- Give your child drinks or food that contain caffeine or sugar before bed
- Participate in playful activity before bedtime

Like younger children, teens are also prone to sleep problems, as highlighted by the 2006 National Sleep Foundation poll. The survey found that, on average, adolescents get about seven and a half hours of sleep on school nights; the amount varies by grade, with teens tending to sleep less as they get older. An estimated 45 percent of adolescents are getting an insufficient amount of sleep on school nights and 31 percent get a borderline amount of sleep (eight to less than nine hours). This means that only 20 percent of adolescents are getting an adequate amount of zzzs. Teens sleeping less on school nights are much more likely to feel sleepy, irritable, and depressed as well as fall asleep in class and drink caffeinated beverages the next day. In addition, adolescents who get insufficient sleep are more likely than their peers to get lower grades. In contrast, the poll found that 71 percent of parents believe their teen gets enough sleep every night or almost every night. (See A Quick Guide to Teens & Sleep on page 141.)

Sleeping as we age

A number of myths surround sleep and aging. *The more birthdays we celebrate, the more sleep we need. As we get older, sleep quality goes downhill. Activity is for kids; naps are for grandparents.*

None of these assumptions are true. Many seniors sleep about the same amount when they are over 65 as they did when they were younger – they just might not sleep those seven to nine hours in the same stretch of time. Some find that the amount of sleep they need to feel refreshed is less than it had once been. And others (the ones who usually go to sleep clinics) are dissatisfied with the change in sleep that occurred with age and are looking for explanations.

Of course, we might nap during the day; our bodies are wired based on circadian rhythms that tend to slow us down in late afternoon. This is normal for all adults. And activity is "just for the kids?" Not so. Active older adults who are engaged socially with family and friends, who are in high spirits, who exercise, and maintain a positive outlook on life will experience less trouble falling asleep at night and fewer nighttime awakenings.

The myth that sleep quality deteriorates with age was debunked by a recent National Sleep Foundation poll, which reported that many older Americans actually sleep better than adults ages 18 to 54. The study showed that 56 percent of older adults (ages 55 to 84) sleep an average of seven to nine hours on weeknights and weekends compared to 51 percent of younger adults.

However, our sleep quality and quantity do change as we age, and it is important to distinguish between what is normal and what symptoms are signs of a sleep disorder.

What is "normal" sleep for mature adults? Just as each of us ages differently, our sleep patterns evolve and change as we grow older. Some go gray sooner or retire into a more sedentary lifestyle, while others are engaged and just as active as their adult children. Some sleep often during the day and report restless nights. Others sleep fitfully, wake up energized, and notice that they need less sleep than they did when they were younger.

We know a number of facts about sleep and aging. Understanding that certain changes are normal can help us distinguish between maturation and the onset of a sleep disorder.

- Older people sleep about the same amount as when they were younger but are less likely to sleep during one stretch of time.

- Mature adults spend the same amount of time in REM sleep but spend less time in deeper stages of NREM sleep.

- Most people over 65 years old wake up more often during the night.

- As we age, our internal sleep clocks, or circadian rhythms, take longer to adjust to changes. This can trigger sleep problems in those who travel frequently or who work irregular hours.

- Because older adults spend less time in deep sleep stages, they tend to be more sensitive to environmental disturbances, such as changes in temperature, light, and outside noise.

- Older adults might have a quiet, restricted lifestyle or sleep often during the day. Less active individuals tend to experience more difficulty sleeping at night simply because they are not as tired.

Typical sleep complaints

Because our sleep quantity and quality changes as we age, older adults often complain of insomnia-related symptoms, such as waking frequently during the night or watching the clock tick for hours before falling asleep.

Sometimes, age-related changes can disguise sleep disorders. About two-thirds of older adults surveyed in 2003 by the National Sleep Foundation say they experience one or more of the following symptoms at least a few nights each week:

- Difficulty falling asleep
- Waking often during the night
- Waking up early and not being able to go back to sleep
- Feeling unrefreshed in the morning
- Snoring
- Pauses in breathing
- Unpleasant feelings in legs

Interestingly, only a fraction of survey respondents with these complaints said they had been diagnosed with a sleep disorder. One thing these older adults did have in common was their health. Eighty-five percent of those who rated their health as only fair or poor reported sleep problems.

Sleep, health, and older adults

A number of factors affect how we sleep when we age; some of them are medical, others are emotional. Less activity and general aches and pains keep some mature adults awake at night. Also, life changes, such as loss of a loved one, can disrupt sleep. When a wife has slept next to her husband for forty years and then must retire to bed at night alone, this difficult life transition will inevitably inhibit sleep.

But poor sleep also is strongly associated with medical and psychiatric problems that may develop as we age. Illnesses can promote sleep disorders. Depression is known to disrupt sleep (and often parlays into insomnia). Chronic obstructive pulmonary disease, heart disease, and arthritis are typical causes of sleep problems. Also, medications can prevent patients from falling or staying asleep, and even alterations in dosage or timing can affect sleep quality.

Conversely, medical problems can disguise primary sleep disorders, and frequent awakenings or daytime sleepiness can be misinterpreted as a side effect of a medical condition. A patient might not respond to treatment for the medical problem, continuing to feel tired, irritable, or restless at night. Rather than considering that these symptoms indicate a primary sleep disorder, the patient simply assumes that he is sick and needs more medication or treatment.

Following are a handful of sleep disorders that present later in life. (These conditions are not limited to mature adults, but are more likely to occur in older individuals than other sleep disorders.)

Sleep apnea

Sleep apnea disrupts breathing to varying degrees in one of four people over the age of 60. Primary symptoms are daytime sleepiness and snoring.

Wandering

Confusion and wandering during the night is common among senior adults who live in long-term care facilities. This situation is a catch-22. Many times, caregivers in hospitals or nursing homes dispense sedative drugs to wanderers so they do not injure themselves or disturb others in the facility. However, some of these drugs further promote confusion and increase the chances of falling. In fact, seniors treated with some sedatives are at an increased risk of hip fractures sustained during nighttime strolls.

Disorientation from taking drugs in the benzodiazepine class can happen outside the nursing home, too. A doctor boarded a plane to South America, where he was slated to speak at an international medical convention. To offset jet lag, he took a benzo pill. But rather than arriving at his destination refreshed and ready for the conference, he accidentally deplaned during a connection when he was supposed to stay on the aircraft. He wandered the airport, completely confused. He was in the wrong country, which he didn't realize until he finally broke down and asked an attendant for help. He did make it to the conference, but he arrived with jet lag, too shaken from the experience to chance taking a benzo again.

Advanced sleep phase syndrome

A pattern of "early to bed, early to rise" can develop as we age. In this case, early might mean well before 9 p.m., in which case rising occurs during hours when most adult are still asleep. Those with advanced sleep phase syndrome might wake up at 4 a.m. after sleeping for seven hours. This sleep schedule can inhibit a person from enjoying a fulfilling social life.

Patients with ASPS should try to stay awake later to postpone early morning awakenings. Exposure to daylight in late afternoon can "trick" the body's internal clock into staying up later.

Periodic limb movement disorder

About one-third of people over 60 experience leg movement like twitching or muscle jerks during the night. Movements that cause arousal can affect the quality of sleep.

REM behavior disorder

Most people who suffer from this disorder are men over 50. Paralysis does not occur during REM sleep, and a person can act out dreams, sometimes resulting in violent physical behavior that harms the patient or his bed partner. (Read more about this in Chapter 10.)

A healthy night's sleep

Sleep hygiene is just as important for mature adults as it is for younger people and children just learning healthy bedtime behavior. Because older individuals are even more sensitive to light, sound, and temperature during sleep, establishing an environment that promotes sleep is especially important.

- Maintain regular bed and wake times
- Go to sleep only when you are drowsy
- Use your bedroom only for sleep and intimate relations

- Avoid excessive daytime naps; if you nap, do so at the same time each day and for no longer than one hour
- Stay active during the day
- Avoid large meals before bed
- Avoid nicotine and caffeine within six hours of bedtime
- Limit alcohol consumption
- Develop a bedtime ritual

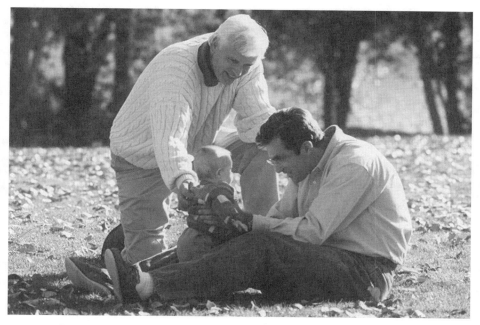

Active days for restful nights

Slowing down when you get older is natural; stopping activity all together will compound sleep and other medical problems. Of course, active is a relative term. For some individuals, a quick walk around the block once a day is enough to tire out the body and promote sleep at night. For others, activity is gardening, visiting with a friend or family member, or going to the store. Activity is also mental: reading, writing a letter, knitting, or completing a crossword puzzle. For less mobile people, active is simply staying awake rather than sleeping through one television program after the next.

Depending on how lively your mental and physical condition allows you to be, some level of activity is essential for maintaining overall health – and for sleeping soundly at night.

Chapter 13

Sleep Medicine Today

*Sleep is the golden chain that ties health
and our bodies together.*

– Thomas Dekker

We are a divided nation – at least that is what the National Sleep Foundation (NSF) discovered in its 2005 Sleep in America poll. Half of us sleep soundly, and the other half, well, we're probably watching more late-night infomercials and counting far too many sheep to get those coveted hours of sleep we need. Meanwhile, troubled sleepers get into 60 percent more automobile accidents and are more likely to be diagnosed with high blood pressure, arthritis, heartburn,

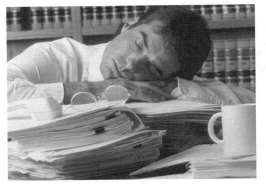

and diabetes than the well-rested bunch. What's more, 64 percent of non-sleepers are overweight, according to the poll. And many non-sleepers are too exhausted and frustrated to perform well at work or to function properly at home.

"[Sleep] is not something to take for granted, ignore, or shortchange," wrote Richard Gelula, CEO of the NSF, in an op-ed article distributed to national newspapers shortly after the 2005 poll results were released. "Rather, sleep is the critical third element, along with diet and exercise, of a healthy, happy lifestyle."

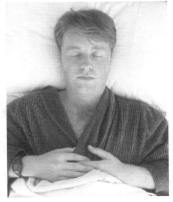

Our health and happiness depend on a good night's sleep, and today, more patients and physicians are recognizing the role sleep medicine plays in promoting overall wellness.

> *... there is a difference between periods of troubled sleep and symptoms of a serious sleep disorder that can have devastating life consequences.*

Attention, please

Once below the radar, sleep medicine is gaining more attention. Advances in research are sparking interest in the field and its relevance to other specialties, from pediatrics to cardiology to bariatric surgery. Sleep medicine is not an isolated island in the medical world – it shares space with every discipline because sleep affects our whole health. A record of disturbed sleep, daytime sleepiness, and problematic sleeping behavior such as snoring worsen pre-existing medical problems and can interfere with treatment.

Sleep medicine plays a critical role in the way doctors treat patients for other medical problems. In fact, a laundry list of diseases are linked to primary sleep disorders:

- Cardiologists are increasingly recognizing that nearly 50 percent of their patients might suffer from sleep apnea.

- Difficulty falling asleep, staying asleep, or early morning awakening is one of the most common presenting symptoms of mood disorders, such as depression or anxiety.

- Strong connections exist between REM behavior disorder and other neurological illnesses such as Parkinson's disease and even post-traumatic stress disorder.

- Restless legs syndrome is common in patients with anemia or low iron, and also in dialysis patients.

- Children with attention deficit disorder are more likely to be diagnosed with obstructive sleep apnea.

- Partial sleep deprivation was recently shown to increase one's risk of developing diabetes.

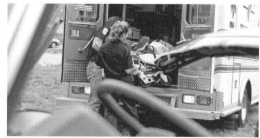

Now more than ever before, sleep specialists identify other health problems when they conduct sleep assessments and interviews. There are also the social issues that arise from disrupted sleep: occupational and motor vehicle accidents; academic underachievement; inability to carry on healthy relationships; and diminished workplace performance.

Making more beds

Once a "luxury" test with a long waiting list, overnight sleep studies are on the rise and becoming more of a norm at medical institutions, which are building these labs and funding sleep medicine departments as patient demand continues to soar. Cleveland Clinic sleep experts test nearly 100 patients each week in one on-site and two off-site lab locations. This is a tremendous jump from just over one year ago, when the one lab housed in the main medical facility tested forty-five patients and the waiting list for an overnight study was six months long.

For the first time ... primary care physicians are realizing that RLS is a disorder that causes sleep loss, and sleep loss is associated with increased occupational hazards and poor health.

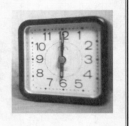

Why the demand? Why all the attention on sleep? And why are patients – and their insurance providers – willing to pay for these tests?

Doctors can point to a media blitz prompted in part by the NSF Sleep in America poll and advances in sleep research, the results of which are reported in consumer magazines and other publications. *Why Aren't You Sleeping? Get More Sleep Tonight! Sleep More, Weigh Less.* These and other headlines directed us to think more seriously about the way sleep affects every part of our lives – not just our energy level during the day, but our risk of crashing our cars, our potential for gaining weight, and our ability to establish and keep lasting relationships.

While doctors conduct more overnight sleep studies in conjunction with medical assessments for an array of health problems, patients ask for polysomnograms, too. The general public understands sleep is important. Not sleeping is a problem – one that we can probably solve if we turn to our doctors for help. The media tell us it's worth our time to catch some zzzs, and national health associations like the NSF are confirming it with reports about how sleep affects our overall health.

Finding an accredited sleep lab

You might think a sleep study is like a chest X-ray – same test, different lab, no big deal. This is not the case. If your doctor recommends a sleep center for your overnight study, you should double-check that the facility is accredited by the American Academy of Sleep Medicine. Some insurance companies will decline coverage for studies that take place in an unaccredited lab, and some labs are accredited as sleep apnea labs only, while others have full accreditation and may be more experienced handling other problems such as narcolepsy, RLS, and nocturnal seizures. Many have limited experience dealing with children.

Sleep Center Resources

Many sleep centers, both affiliated with medical centers and independent, have websites that describe the services they offer. Here are some places to start:

American Academy of Sleep Medicine
www.aasmnet.org

American Insomnia Association
www.americaninsomniaassociation.org

American Sleep Apnea Association
www.sleepapnea.org

Cleveland Clinic Sleep Disorders Center
www.clevelandclinic.org/neuroscience/treat/sleep/

Narcolepsy Network
www.websciences.org/narnet

National Institutes of Health
www.nih.gov

National Sleep Foundation
www.sleepfoundation.org

Restless Legs Syndrome Foundation
www.rls.org

Sleep Research Society
www.sleepresearchsociety.org

Insurance coverage and your sleep study

In general, coverage for overnight sleep studies is not a problem for patients with sleep apnea and narcolepsy because both disorders are widely recognized as having adverse affects on health and performance. They are treatable and can be readily diagnosed with an overnight sleep test.

More often, insurance providers take a second look at claims that request coverage for an overnight sleep study to diagnose insomnia, the most common sleep complaint. Most people with insomnia need a detailed sleep and medical history, not necessarily an overnight sleep study. Only in severe cases in which sleep assessments and clinical testing have failed will sleep specialists order an overnight test for insomnia patients. The majority of insomnia cases can be treated with medications and behavioral therapy.

> *Why the demand? Why all the attention on sleep?*
> *And why are patients – and their insurance providers –*
> *willing to invest in sleep evaluations?*

Beyond overnight sleep studies, insurance companies cover treatments such as continuous positive airway pressure therapy (when a patient is diagnosed with obstructive sleep apnea by an overnight sleep study); certain medications; dental devices (though this depends on provider and diagnosis); and specific, approved surgeries. Coverage always varies with provider and region.

New treatments

As our society tunes in to the importance of getting a good night's sleep, physicians and researchers are discovering new treatments and multiple uses for drugs already on the market. For example, modafinil, prescribed for narcolepsy, is now approved to treat hypersomnia in obstructive sleep apnea and shift work sleep disorder. Requip (ropinirole) is the only drug approved by the Food and Drug Administration for treatment of restless legs syndrome, and a media blast educating consumers on the drug is also sparking awareness of RLS.

In the non-benzodiazepine hypnotics category, Ambien and Sonata were introduced to the market, followed in 2005 by Lunesta. All are designed to help insomniacs rest easy. Lunesta is the only hypnotic to date approved for long-term use. Approved by the FDA in 2005, Rozerem is the first prescription insomnia medication that targets the normal sleep-wake cycle. It is a melatonin receptor agonist, and it's the first drug that does not act by depressing the central nervous system. It is also the first drug for insomnia without abuse potential.

The rapidly growing interest in sleep medicine among the pharmaceutical community is advancing the ways physicians can treat sleep disorders. Today there are simply more pharmaceutical options. This trend shows no sign of slowing.

> *With sleep, there simply is no standard. Sleep changes as we age, as our bodies progress through various stages in our lives, and as we experience emotions that inevitably take a toll on our sleep quality.*

No substitute for sleep

A good night's sleep varies from person to person. Seven hours of sleep is a luxury to one person while nine hours is more suitable for another. With sleep, there simply is no standard. It changes as we age, as our bodies progress through various stages in our lives, and as we experience emotions that inevitably take a toll on our sleep quality.

But there is a difference between periods of troubled sleep and symptoms of a serious sleep disorder. If daytime sleepiness, forgetfulness, irritability, or restless nights are concerns for you, it's important to talk to your doctor, who will determine whether your patterns are cause for concern.

Our bodies are wired differently and our chemistry is unique and complex. And no, there isn't a single formula for sound sleep. Perhaps this is why we marvel over

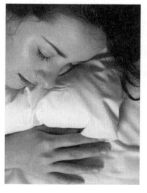

sleep – no matter how much we know, quite a bit remains a mystery. But as we now can identify "normal sleep" in a scientific sense, we can determine patterns in patients who display abnormal sleep behavior. We can diagnose and treat sleep disorders – and we can improve our overall health because of it. Sleep isn't a waste of time. Your health today and tomorrow vitally depends on it. Your awareness of its role in your path to wellness is the first step toward a lifetime of true good nights.

Appendix 1

The Sleep Lab Experience: Questions and Answers

Sweet Dreams in the Sleep Lab

If you struggle to get a good night's sleep, the thought of checking into a medical facility and tucking into a strange bed in a sterile environment doesn't seem like any way to rest easy. Add the wires, monitors, and hardware essential to recording your sleep patterns – as if you will sleep – and you're as likely to doze off in the sleep lab as in the dentist's chair during a root canal, right? Who signed you up for this gig anyway?!

Never fear. Though a bit awkward and not as comfortable as your own bed, virtually everyone falls asleep during an overnight study. (Anyway, you are probably so exhausted that even if you think you won't catch a wink, your body will be thankful for a sleep-friendly environment.)

And as for the wires – those are actually fairly non-invasive. Yes, you will feel a bit different with eight sensors on your head, five spread on your chest and legs, and a couple of tubes near your nostrils. You might even feel electric – wired for sleep, one might say. But as a technologist prepares you for the study, explaining each sensor and the purpose of these devices, you will soon realize that they are not restrictive and are critical to helping you sleep better in the future.

As you prepare for your first overnight sleep study, let's cover some questions that might cross your mind.

What should I do before the test? Can I go out to dinner with my spouse? What about my morning coffee?

If you support a vicious coffee habit, you should pare down to a morning cup. Your study will not begin until your normal bedtime, so there is no reason to avoid caffeine completely, as long as you cut it off before mid-afternoon. Sure – go out to dinner, and go about your day as you normally would. Just avoid nicotine, alcohol, and excessive exercise that might keep you awake longer than otherwise.

Will I be able to go to work the next day?

That depends on whether you need to stay for a nap test. The multiple sleep latency test will require you to stay at the lab throughout the day. In between nap trials, you will have down-time to read, work on a laptop, or participate in another low-key activity. A technologist will set the stage for a nap – dimming lights, asking you to lie down and shut your eyes – every so often. Many labs will provide breakfast and lunch, but ask about this in advance.

Be sure to tell the technologist about your plans for the next day or whether you require a certain wake-up time. If you are scheduled for an MSLT, you should plan on taking the day off work. In most sleep centers, the sleep rooms are equipped with showers so you can go directly to work if you're free to leave after the overnight recording.

What will the doctor learn from my study?

If the overnight sleep study was successful, your doctor will be able to diagnose a sleep disorder if you have one. One of the most common reasons patients endure overnight sleep studies is to diagnose sleep apnea. Such diagnoses usually can be made after a one-night stay at the lab.

How will technologists gather all of this information?

By fixing sensors to your head, chest, abdomen, and legs, a technologist will measure a number of activities while you sleep. A pulse oximeter probe measures your oxygen level, and a couple of sensors placed by the nostrils and outside the mouth record breathing patterns. During the night, a technologist will record: eye movement; sleep staging (when your body enters stages 1 through 4 and REM); leg movements; heart rate; respiration; oxygen; body position; and snoring (through a snore microphone). Do not be alarmed if your study is videotaped; this is an important part of the study, as technologists can watch body position-ing as it relates to sleep disturbances. Your technologist will notify you of this in advance.

Will I really fall asleep with all of those sensors? I'm not used to being in a strange bed – and I'm kind of freaked out by hospital environments.

There is such a thing as first-night effect, when patients do not sleep well because they are too disturbed by the foreign environment. But in most cases, patients sleep much longer than they think. After the study, a technologist will ask you to estimate how long you slept. When compared with actual time recorded, patients usually low-ball their responses.

As for sleeping with sensors, again, most patients are so exhausted, sleep-deprived, and actually craving an environment that fosters sound sleep that they do not have a problem once they adjust to the feeling of having some extra "hardware" in bed with them.

And today, most sleep labs do not have the ambience of a hospital, even those housed in medical facilities. Rooms are much like hotel rooms, often with private bathrooms, televisions, and other amenities. Some sleep medicine clinics are actually moving into wings of hotels and converting rooms into sleep testing centers. This is especially appealing to patients who feel uncomfortable about sleeping overnight at a hospital.

I'm used to sleeping with my spouse. Can someone come with me?

Unless you need your spouse to assist you with functions like going to the rest-room in the middle of the night, the sleep lab is reserved only for patients. A parent or significant other must be present if the patient is under 18 years old. Pullout sofas are available in the lab rooms for guests.

Appendix 2

Most Commonly Used Sleep Aids at drugstore.com*

Active Ingredients	Brand names
Acetaminophen and diphenhydramine hydrochloride	Extra Strength Acetaminophen PM®; Extra Strength PM®; Legatrin PM®
Acetaminophen and diphenhydramine citrate	Excedrin PM®
Aspirin and diphenhydramine citrate	Alka-Seltzer PM®; Bayer NightTime Relief®
Diphenhydramine hydrochloride	GoodNight's Sleep®; Nytol®; Simply sleep®; Sominex®; Unisom sleep gel®
Diphenhydramine hydrochloride and magnesium salicylate tetrahydrate	Doan's PM®
Doxylamine succinate	Unisom Night Time Sleep Aid®
Hyoscyamus Niger, nux Moschata, Passiflora Incarnata, Robinia Pseudoacacia, Stramonium	Boiron Quietude®
Natrum Muriaticum, Lycopodium, Ignatia, Valeriana, Chamomilla, etc	Moon Drops®
Passiflora incarnata (Passion Flower), avena sativa, Humulus lupulus	Hylands Calms Forte®
St. Ignatius' bean, sea salt, kava-kava, etc.	NaturalCare Anxiety Relief®

* As reported in Recent Advances in the Treatment of Insomnia, by Kumar Budur, M.D., Carlos Rodriguez, M.D., and Nancy Foldvary-Schaefer, D.O., Cleveland Clinic Journal of Medicine, 2006.

Appendix 3

Beck Depression Inventory

On this questionnaire are groups of statements. Please read each group of statements carefully, then pick out the one statement in each group which best describes the way that you have been feeling in the past week, including today. Mark the square beside the statement you picked. If several statements in the group seem to apply equally well, mark each one. Be sure to read all the statements in each group before making your choice.

1. ☐ 0 I do not feel sad
   ☐ 1 I feel sad
   ☐ 2 I am sad all the time and I can't snap out of it
   ☐ 3 I am so sad or unhappy that I can't stand it

2. ☐ 0 I am not particularly discouraged about the future
   ☐ 1 I feel discouraged about the future
   ☐ 2 I feel I have nothing to look forward to
   ☐ 3 I feel the future is hopeless and cannot improve

3. ☐ 0 I do not feel like a failure
   ☐ 1 I feel I have failed more than the average person
   ☐ 2 As I look back on my life I see lots of failures
   ☐ 3 I feel I am a complete failure as a person

4. ☐ 0 I get as much satisfaction out of things as I used to
   ☐ 1 I don't enjoy things the way I used to
   ☐ 2 I don't get real satisfaction out of anything anymore
   ☐ 3 I am dissatisfied or bored with everything

5. ☐ 0 I don't feel particularly guilty
   ☐ 1 I feel guilty a good part of the time
   ☐ 2 I feel guilty most of the time
   ☐ 3 I feel guilty all of the time

6. ❑ 0 I don't feel I am being punished
   ❑ 1 I feel I may be punished
   ❑ 2 I expect to be punished
   ❑ 3 I feel I am being punished

7. ❑ 0 I don't feel disappointed in myself
   ❑ 1 I am disappointed in myself
   ❑ 2 I am disgusted with myself
   ❑ 3 I hate myself

8. ❑ 0 I don't feel I am any worse than anybody else
   ❑ 1 I am critical of myself for my weaknesses and mistakes
   ❑ 2 I blame myself all of the time for my faults
   ❑ 3 I blame myself for everything bad that happens

9. ❑ 0 I don't have any thoughts of killing myself
   ❑ 1 I have thoughts of killing myself but would not carry them out
   ❑ 2 I would like to kill myself
   ❑ 3 I would kill myself if I had the chance

10. ❑ 0 I don't cry any more than usual
    ❑ 1 I cry more than I used to
    ❑ 2 I used to be able to cry
    ❑ 3 I used to be able to cry, but now I can't cry even though I want to

11. ❑ 0 I am no more irritated now than I ever am
    ❑ 1 I get annoyed or irritated more easily than I used to
    ❑ 2 I feel irritated all the time now
    ❑ 3 I don't get irritated at all by the things that used to irritate me

12. ❑ 0 I have not lost interest in other people
    ❑ 1 I'm less interested in other people than I used to be
    ❑ 2 I have lost most of my interest in other people
    ❑ 3 I have lost all of my interest in other people

13. ❑ 0 I make decisions about as well as I ever could
    ❑ 1 I put off making decisions more than I used to
    ❑ 2 I have greater difficulty in making decisions than before
    ❑ 3 I can't make decisions at all anymore

14. ❑ 0 I don't feel I look worse than I used to
    ❑ 1 I am worried that I look old or unattractive
    ❑ 2 I feel that there are permanent changes in my appearance
    ❑ 3 I feel that there are permanent changes in my appearance that make
        me look unattractive

15. ❑ 0 I can work about as well as before
    ❑ 1 It takes an extra effort to get started doing something
    ❑ 2 I have to push myself very hard to do anything
    ❑ 3 I can't do any work at all

16. ❑ 0 I can sleep as well as usual
    ❑ 1 I don't sleep as well as I used to
    ❑ 2 I wake up 1 to 2 hours earlier than I used to and find it hard
        to get back to sleep
    ❑ 3 I wake up several hours earlier than I used to and cannot get
        back to sleep

17. ❑ 0 I don't get more tired than usual
    ❑ 1 I get tired more easily than I used to
    ❑ 2 I get tired from doing almost anything
    ❑ 3 I am too tired to do anything

18. ❑ 0 My appetite is no worse than usual
    ❑ 1 My appetite is not as good as it used to be
    ❑ 2 My appetite is much worse now
    ❑ 3 I have no appetite at all anymore

19. ❑ 0 I haven't lost much weight, if any, lately
    ❑ 1 I have lost more than 5 pounds. I am purposely trying to lose weight
    ❑ 2 I have lost more than 10 pounds by eating less
    ❑ 3 I have lost more than 15 pounds

20. ❏ 0 I am no more worried about my health than usual
    ❏ 1 I am worried about physical problems such as aches and
        pains or upset stomach and constipation
    ❏ 2 I am very worried about physical problems and it's hard to
        think of much else
    ❏ 3 I am so worried about my physical problems that I cannot
        think of anything else

21. ❏ 0 I have not noticed any recent change in my interest in sex
    ❏ 1 I am less interested in sex than I used to be
    ❏ 2 I am much less interested in sex now
    ❏ 3 I have lost interest in sex completely

Index

A

B

I

J

K

L

M

R

S

A Quick Guide to Getting a Good Night's Sleep

Sleep rejuvenates the body so it can function properly during waking hours. That's reason enough to do everything possible to ensure an adequate amount of quality zzzzs. Here are some tips:

Use your bedroom only for sleep and intimate relations.

This means:

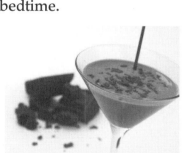

- Not watching television or even reading in bed;

- Not eating in bed;

- Definitely not working in bed.

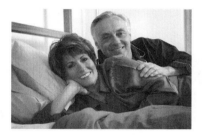

Essentially, you want to make your bedroom a calming oasis. Even an alarm clock can be a distraction. Try facing it away from you so that you don't obsess about the time while you're trying to fall asleep.

Avoid caffeine within four to six hours of bedtime.

This includes:

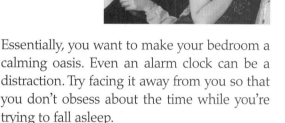

- Coffee, tea, and soda;

- Chocolate;

- Over-the-counter wakefulness-promoting agents and some prescription drugs.

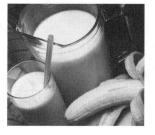

If you suffer from insomnia, limit caffeinated beverages and avoid drinking caffeine after noon. Excessive caffeine use can lead to withdrawal symptoms, which can affect one's ability to sleep.

Avoid nicotine close to bedtime

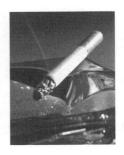

Like caffeine, nicotine is a sleep-inhibiting stimulant. Smokers who break the habit might experience withdrawal symptoms at first, but once their body adjusts, they will find that they wake up less and sleep more soundly at night. If you can't quit the habit entirely, avoid smoking in the evening and absolutely during the night.

Do not drink alcoholic beverages within four to six hours of bedtime

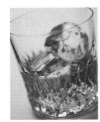

Despite the notion that a "nightcap" is just the thing for a good night's sleep, alcoholic beverages actually interfere with the body's ability to maintain deep sleep, which refreshes the body. Alcohol might induce sleep at first, but regular users are likely to wake up frequently and often report feeling drowsy and sleep deprived in the morning.

Avoid large meals; settle for a small snack before bedtime.

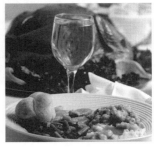

Full meals before bedtime can trigger heartburn and stomachache – two reasons to eat heavy meals no later than four hours before going to sleep. A light snack, on the other hand, can promote sleep. Milk or cheese and crackers are good bedtime snacks.

In addition:

• Sleep only when you are drowsy.

• If you cannot fall or stay asleep, leave your bedroom and read or engage in a relaxing activity in another room.

• Do not allow yourself to fall asleep outside the bedroom; return to the bed to rest.

• Maintain regular bed and wake times.

• Avoid napping during the day. (If you're extremely exhausted, limit naps to less than one hour, no later than 3 p.m.)

• Avoid strenuous exercise within six hours of going go to sleep.

• Minimize light, noise, and extreme temperatures in the bedroom.

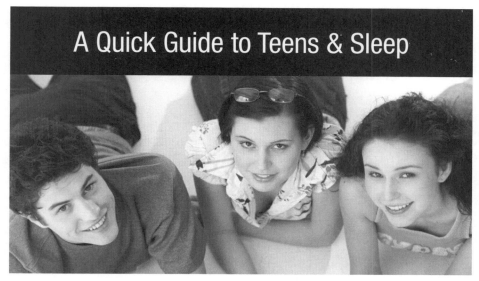

A Quick Guide to Teens & Sleep

The National Sleep Foundation's 2006 Sleep in America poll focused on the sleep habits of America's adolescents (sixth- to twelfth-graders). It found that teens are not getting the sleep they need, and this lack of sleep gets worse as they progress through their teen years.

For parents, here's how to help your teens on the road to good nights and better mornings:

1) Set a consistent bedtime and wake-time for your teen (even on weekends) that allows for at least 8.5-9.25 hours of sleep each night.

2) Encourage your teen to establish a relaxing bedtime routine that includes pleasure reading, taking a bath, or listening to music.

3) Set up a bedroom for your teen that is cool, dark, and quiet.

4) Keep the television, computer, and cell phone in the living room or den instead of your teen's bedroom – these high-tech gadgets are often "sleep stealers."

5) Help your teen to cut out caffeine after lunchtime.

6) Create an environment that allows your teen to get into bright light in the morning and avoid it in the evening.

7) Be a good role model – talk to your teen about the importance of sleep and set the tone by making sleep a priority in your life.

Used with permission of the National Sleep Foundation. For further information, please visit http://www.sleepfoundation.org.

For teens, here are some sleep-smart tips:

1) **Sleep is food for the brain:** Get enough of it, and get it when you need it. Even mild sleepiness can hurt your performance – from taking school exams to playing sports or video games. Lack of sleep can make you look tired and feel depressed, irritable, and angry.

2) **Keep consistency in mind:** Establish a regular bedtime and wake-time schedule and maintain it during weekends and school (or work) vacations. Don't stray from your schedule frequently and never do so for two or more consecutive nights. If you must go off schedule, avoid delaying your bedtime by more than one hour, awaken the next day within two hours of your regular schedule, and, if you are sleepy during the day, take an early afternoon nap.

3) **Learn how much sleep you need to function at your best.** You should awaken refreshed, not tired. Most adolescents need between 8.5 and 9.5 hours of sleep each night. Know when you need to get up in the morning, then calculate when you need to go to sleep to get at least 8.5 hours of sleep a night.

4) **Get into bright light as soon as possible in the morning, but avoid it in the evening.** The light helps to signal to the brain when it should wake up and when it should prepare to sleep.

5) **Understand your circadian rhythm.** Then you can try to maximize your schedule throughout the day according to your internal clock. For example, to compensate for your "slump (sleepy) times," participate in stimulating activities or classes that are interactive, and avoid lecture classes or potentially unsafe activities, including driving.

6) **After lunch (or after noon), stay away from coffee, colas with caffeine, and nicotine, which are all stimulants.** Also avoid alcohol and recreational drugs, which disrupt sleep and impair daytime functioning.

7) **Relax before going to bed.** Avoid heavy reading, studying, and computer games within one hour of going to bed. Don't fall asleep with the television on – flickering light and stimulating content can inhibit restful sleep. If you work during the week, try to avoid working night hours. If you work until 9:30 p.m., for example, you will still need to plan time to unwind before going to sleep.

8) **Say no to all-nighters.** Staying up late can cause chaos to your sleep patterns and your ability to be alert the next day – and beyond. Remember, the best thing you can do to prepare for a test is to get plenty of sleep. All-nighters or late-night study sessions might seem to give you more time to cram for your exam, but they are also likely to drain your brainpower.

Used with permission of the National Sleep Foundation. For further information, please visit http://www.sleepfoundation.org.

A Quick Guide to Sleep & Certain Conditions

How to get a good night's sleep when you have:

Obstructive sleep apnea.

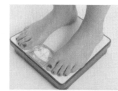

• Lose weight. Even moderate weight loss can improve breathing during sleep.

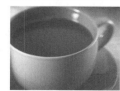

• Avoid alcohol and central nervous system depressants before bed.

• Change your sleeping position. Some patients exhibit OSA only when they sleep on their backs. A side sleeping position is known to reduce apneic episodes.

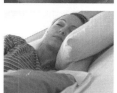

• Take medication for nasal congestion. Those with sinus problems or frequent nasal congestion are more likely to experience OSA.

Restless legs syndrome.

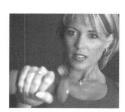

• Exercise regularly. A regular exercise program can reduce symptoms of RLS in patients with mild cases.

• Reduce caffeine intake.

• Limit use of alcohol.

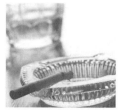

• Stop smoking.

• Eliminate drugs known to cause RLS.

• Walk, ride an exercise bike, massage lower leg area, or soak in a hot tub to help alleviate leg sensations.

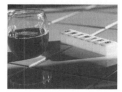

Since iron deficiency is a reversible cause of RLS, many sleep specialists recommend over-the-counter iron tablets (ferrous sulfate). A simple blood test can measure iron stores in the body and help physicians determine who might benefit from iron therapy.

Sleep terrors.

When your child suffers from sleep terrors:

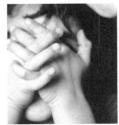

• Do not try to yell, coax, or shake a child out of a sleep terror. During this deep sleep stage, the child is having an incomplete arousal; this means he or she is still technically asleep yet able to move and appears awake.

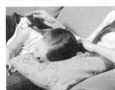

• On the other hand, young children will unknowingly appreciate a hug and comforting touch. Though they will probably not respond to comforting actions, holding a child is a natural and healthy reaction to sleep terrors.

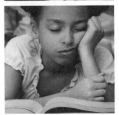

• Because exhaustion and stress can spur sleep terrors, ensure that your child gets enough rest. Normal routines foster healthy sleep habits, and your child's activities during the day will have an impact on his or her ability to sleep soundly.

Narcolepsy.

If you suffer from excessive daytime sleepiness, you may want to consider one of these commonly prescribed stimulants:

• Ritalin

• Adderall

• Concerta

• Dexedrine

• Focalin

• Metadate

Delayed sleep-phase syndrome.

• Practice good sleep hygiene.

• Ask your physician about prescribing melatonin or light therapy.